Shocking Stories of Nursing:

Memoirs Of A 50-Year Nursing Career

Laura A. Conklin,
MSN, MSA, RN

COPYRIGHT

Shocking Stories of Nursing: Memoirs of a 50-year Nursing Career
Copyright 2020 by Laura A. Conklin

Layout by Douglas Williams
Editorial support by Pat Iyer

Published by:
Nurlewood Publishing, LLC
21718 Edgewood Street
St. Clair Shores, MI 48080
586-596-5239

A great gift for a nurse, student nurse, or someone interested in a healthcare career. The stories are real. Some are hilarious, some are tragic, but all are designed to give the reader a glimpse behind the curtain of secrecy that sometimes veils the mysterious world of healthcare. An inspirational look into my rewarding and dedicated career in nursing. You will be entertained!

ISBN: 9798666480748

Acknowledgment

First and foremost, I want to thank Pat Iyer for mentoring me through this process. This book also would not have been possible without the encouragement of my family: my husband Ronald (deceased) and my twin sister Loretta (deceased), my son Ryan, my daughter Hollie and her husband Tony, my grandsons Jake and Max, and many friends. They told me, "You've got to write a book!" A special thank you to Sue, the world's best neighbor and her twin sister Patty; and Marie, Delores, Andrea, and Vivian, for reading the drafts and their support. I can't forget to acknowledge George and Margie for their hospitality and providing me with a peaceful environment in which to gather my thoughts and Elaine, the inspiration for my career in nursing.

About the Author

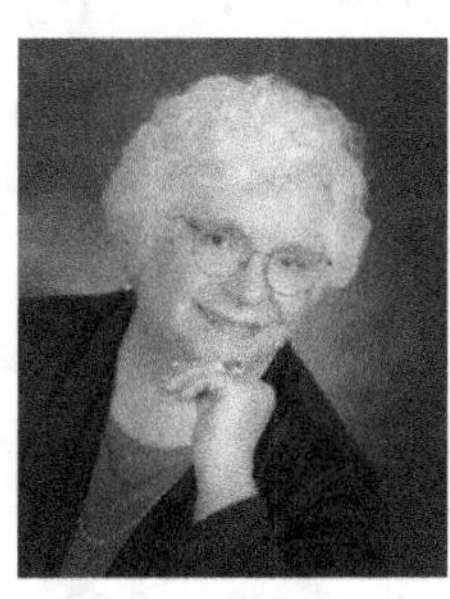

Laura has an extensive and distinguished nursing career. She is a graduate of Mercy College of Detroit (UD-Mercy), Central Michigan University, and the University of Phoenix. Ms. Conklin also completed studies in clinical wound healing at The Page and William Black Postgraduate School of Mount Sinai School of Medicine, Tufts University School of Medicine, and has taken courses at the Wharton School University of Pennsylvania. She is board certified in Orthopedics, Legal Nurse Consulting, Nursing Education and is president of Conklin and Associates, LLC where she assists plaintiff and defense attorneys in the litigation process as a nursing expert. Past certifications include Wound Care, a Fellow in the College of Certified Wound Specialists, and a Diplomate of the American Academy of Wound Management.

She has many publications, seminars, and continuing education sessions listed on her curriculum vitae. Ms. Conklin retired as a Professor of Nursing in 2019 from Wayne County Community College District, having educated and mentored students at various levels and served as an ambassador to the National League for Nursing. Ms. Conklin has published several articles and is a contributing author in D. Ignatavicus & M. Workman's *Medical-Surgical nursing: Critical thinking for collaborative care* (6th ed.) and a chapter author in *Legal nurse consulting practices* (3rd ed.) American Association of Legal Nurse Consultants. In addition, she served as an expert witness for the Bureau of Health Professions of the Michigan Department of Licensing and Regulatory Affairs; and was a consulting expert for the Michigan Department of the Attorney General. Ms. Conklin has presented at numerous conferences (local, national, and international) on various aspects of nursing practice and is an active member of several professional associations.

As a nurse we have the opportunity to heal the mind, soul, heart, and body of our patients, their families and ourselves.

"I've learned that people will forget what you have said, people will forget what you did, but people will never forget how you made them feel."

— Maya Angelou

Contents

Introduction

Have you ever been a patient in the hospital or visited someone? Does the thought of being a patient terrify you? Maybe it should! In this book, you will find unforgettable stories gathered during my 50-year successful nursing career. I have worked in almost every field of nursing and want to share those experiences and stories. I learned a lot; I contributed a lot and moved on to the next adventure. These are my memoirs.

Whether you are interested in what nurses do, are an experienced nurse, or in the healthcare field, you will find this book entertaining. Be prepared to be amused, surprised, and even shocked. All the stories are true. However, the names of individuals and organizations have been changed to protect the innocent, the guilty, the brainless, and those whose names I just absolutely forgot. Some of the stories are outrageous, some are humorous, while others portray humanity at its best and its worst. All are designed to give you a glimpse behind the curtain of secrecy that sometimes veils

the mysterious world of health care. Welcome to
my world!

CHAPTER ONE:

THE EARLY DAYS

"You don't have to be great to start,
but you have to start to be great."

—Zig Ziglar

WHY I WANTED TO BECOME A NURSE

EVER SINCE I can remember I enjoyed helping people and animals. I was the one who found the right size Band-Aid and made sure all booboos were appropriately treated no matter how small or how big. Most of my dolls had bandages. Even the family dog did not escape my tender loving care. Although I must admit removing an adhesive bandage off a hairy dog was a little challenging at times, the patient was not always appreciative nor cooperative. Little did I know in my future I would also encounter some less than cooperative patients who growled occasionally.

I watched medical theme-based movies such as those featuring Dr. Kildare and science fiction ones with the mad scientist creating a cure for something in the basement laboratory. Biographies of famous scientists fascinated me. I liked Frankenstein. The premise was interesting, but the execution was challenging at best. Imagine if he had Crazy Glue what he could accomplish. The monster was an exciting piece of work— amazing what you can do with leftovers and parts if you have some talent.

My godfather's daughter, Elaine, was my inspiration. Elaine was a nurse. I was impressed by how she looked in her starched white uniform, nursing cap, and blue cape, which signified the essence of dedication to suffering humanity. All Elaine needed was wings, and she would be an angel. That's a stretch, but she looked so professional and I wanted to share that image. Whenever we visited her parents, I would sneak into Elaine's bedroom to try on her nursing cap and pretend that I was a nurse. I had a long way to go before I stepped into that role. I had my dreams, and I knew that someday they would come true.

My dad was a butcher who owned a small grocery store. My mother used to tell people he was a surgeon; sometimes, she left out a "pig" surgeon. Being around my dad in the store made me familiar with the sight of blood and guts, muscles, and bones, which was great preparation for being a nurse. Little did I know that my anatomy lessons had begun.

Dad frequently cut himself and needed help with bandages, and I was there with the tape and make sure everything was OK, even though I was still in grade school. Dad was Army tough. Quite often, he cut himself, finished the day's work, then went to the emergency room to get stitches, sometimes too late. Meanwhile, he would just use a little bit of duct tape, or whatever was handy and sometimes that worked better than the stitches. Amazingly he never got an infection. Dad was always good at hand washing.

I lived in a small house with my grandparents, my parents, and my twin sister Loretta. I was always fascinated with the workings of the human anatomy and why things work the way they do or don't. When Loretta was sick, even with a cold or something simple, I would take care of her. She was my baby sister due to my arrival five minutes before her. I swear she pushed me out first with a directive to "check it out, let me know if it's safe to come out". In those days, the father was not allowed in the delivery room. The doctor came out and announced to my dad that he didn't have a son, and he didn't have a daughter. My dad was a little confused until he found out he had two daughters. That might be why I have no more brothers and sisters since if they started coming two at a time, that could be a little scary.

New Sheets Make Great Bandages

At the tender age of six, Loretta was my first victim of Nursing 101. My mother and a group of her lady friends would occasionally gather on the weekend and sew bandages for the Red Cross for the Korean War effort. They would chat, enjoy telling jokes, and make big bandages that were shipped off through the Red Cross for the soldiers.

My mother's American Red Cross First Aid Textbook has fascinating information with lots of pretty pictures on what to do in case of emergencies. One chapter described the appropriate bandaging techniques for all kinds of wounds, along with outstanding pictures and diagrams. That whet my appetite; I couldn't resist. So, while the ladies were busy in the kitchen making bandages, I decided I could do the same thing and practice for my future role as a great nurse. I took one of my mother's brand-new bedsheet (because after all bandages must be clean), and a pair of scissors and made elegant little strips approximately 3-4 inches wide. Then I bandaged Loretta from head to toe following the excellent directions and illustrations the American Red

Cross provided in their First Aid Textbook. Loretta was a somewhat reluctant guinea pig. Once I got the first good bandages in place, she had no choice; she couldn't move. I was impressed. I did a fantastic job!

I must have achieved a remarkable piece of work because when my grandfather came home and saw my handiwork, he thought Loretta had been in a terrible accident. He shouted, "Why didn't you call me?" He soon found out there was no blood, just the enthusiastic results of a future nurse. However, my mother didn't agree. In fact, she left me with the impression that I would be the next one in bandages if I ever tried to do that again. I held on to those dreams and passion. I learned to curb that enthusiasm and not rip up any more practice bandages. Now, if only others could see my talent, I was on my way!

CHAPTER TWO

FROM CANDY STRIPER TO STUDENT NURSE

"Devote yourself. Make it happen. You will struggle. You will overcome your fears! Smile, don't forget this is your dream!"

—Anonymous

As THE YEARS went on, I continued to read stories of nurses and their heroism. I watched any movie or TV drama with a medical theme such as *Dr. Kildare* (1961-1966) portrayed by Richard Chamberlain. (Today that gorgeous doctor would be Matthew McConaughey or Channing Tatum). *Ben Casey, MD*-neurosurgeon (1961-1966), was played by Vincent Edwards (a former "Doctor Dreamy" borrowing the title from Patrick Dempsey of *Grey's Anatomy* fame).

While these shows mostly focused on the drama around the medical profession, there were a lot of nurses in their starched white uniforms and nursing caps assisting the physicians in eliminating human suffering. TV drama showed them flirting and trying to get a doctor to marry them; however, it appeared they participated in the healing efforts at the most crucial times. The doctors couldn't succeed without the nurses being their eyes and ears 24/7 at the bedside. They cared for the patients, continually assessing for and reporting changes in signs and symptoms. All this took place while diligently working together with the physician to cure disease. The nursing roles were exciting but the doctors, Richard Chamberlain, and Vincent Edwards were far more exciting! They were handsome and dedicated. It was occasionally difficult to determine what they were dedicated to, nevertheless, the shows were inspiring.

FUTURE NURSES CLUB AND BEYOND

While in high school, I was an active member of the Future Nurses Club. We discussed schools of nursing, education options, as well as various roles for nurses, which were limited compared to today. The school offered a program through the American Red Cross for anyone interested in a healthcare career to work as a Candy Striper visiting patients in the hospital and assisting nurses with various tasks. When I remembered the bandages and the efforts of the American Red Cross to help those in need, I couldn't resist. I had to be part of this endeavor. Elaine agreed it was a good idea to get involved.

My volunteer destination was a small community hospital in our town, St. Raphael. I had a uniform consisting of a red and white pin-striped pinafore with the Red Cross emblem on the front bib. I also had a nursing cap, the same color as the pinafore, bearing the Red Cross emblem. It wasn't white, but at least it was a nursing cap and made me feel like a nurse. Here I am world; I am ready to help.

The job was simple. As a Candy Striper, I was assigned to a post-operative female unit. I provided patients with fresh water, put fresh flowers in vases, and threw out dead ones. Somehow dead flowers in a patient's room just did not look welcoming or encouraging. They might make the patient wonder, "Am I next?"

Also, I read mail to the patients and visited those who had no visitors. I ran errands and fetched supplies for the nurses. Just being in the environment and observing the activities would help me decide if a healthcare career was for me. No problem, I flourished in this environment and enjoyed the activity.

I wanted to be more involved in the action and wouldn't settle for just passing water and reading get-well cards. I requested a transfer to the Emergency Room (ER)/Central Supply, where the patient encounters were always changing. I felt my talent would be more appreciated; after all I already knew how to make bandages.

The ER consisted of a one room trauma area with an adjacent central supply, well-stocked with everything you might need for a small community hospital. Ms. Mary Aspen managed the area. Although Ms. Aspen was considered by some to be prim and proper, others thought of her as being too strict, but all would agree that she was a dedicated nurse.

Ms. Aspen was a perfectionist: there was only one way to do something and that was *her* way. I learned so much from her regarding prioritizing and time management. I quickly anticipated what supplies were needed for any emergency room visitor. She taught me critical thinking and to foresee both the patient's and doctor's needs. "Plan ahead" was her motto. After all, it wasn't raining when Noah built the ark.

Full moons bring out some of the weirdos in any community. She often said when you're ready for a disaster, it probably won't happen, and, if it does, it won't be a disaster. Our town was no exception; we had our share of quirky patients doing stupid things. One such example was a gentleman who decided to adjust his chainsaw while it was running. Fortunately, he managed to keep all his body parts, however, he did end up with some very nasty lacerations. Another busy mom turned on her gas stove and went looking for a match to light the pilot. When she struck it, she sustained some significant burns on her face losing her eyebrows and some of her hair.

We were ready for just about anything. In today's healthcare world, things have changed dramatically in preparation to meet any emergency. It took a lot of hands-on effort to be ready and have all supplies available for use when needed. Here are a few examples of what those preparations consisted of many years ago.

Only Surgeons Wore Gloves

Before the days of universal precautions and everybody protecting themselves from the spread of potentially dangerous diseases, only surgeons wore gloves. Those gloves had to be washed, hung on racks, turned inside out after one side dried, and then placed back on racks to dry side two. Next, the gloves were placed in a tin with very fine cornstarch and shaken to coat them so they could slip on easily. (I often wondered what that fine powder did to nurses' lungs.) The gloves then had to be folded in a certain way with the right hand on the right side and the left hand on the left side with the sizes matching. They were wrapped in autoclavable paper. The nurse wrote the size of the glove on the paper and then autoclaved them. I often wondered if surgeons wore gloves so as not to leave fingerprints in the patients because the rest of us just frequently washed our hands.

Don't Let the Water Overflow

The autoclave was not just for sterilizing. It had another function – to create distilled water from the steam, which we put into large, heavy glass bottles to provide sterile water for various procedures in the hospital. It took about 5 to 6 minutes to fill the bottle, and you would move the hose from one bottle to the next one until all the bottles were filled. If your time management was a bit off, the water would overrun onto the floor, where you had another job of cleaning it up. Either your time management improved, or you suffered the wrath of Ms. Aspen. Once we capped the bottles, we put the rack of bottles into the autoclave to be sterilized and ready for use. All this took place between seeing patients and performing other duties of the emergency room/central supply area.

Needles and Glass Syringes

The next interesting task was to sharpen the needles used for injections. Yes, the needles needed to be sharpened. There were no prepackaged disposable syringes you could open, use once, and throw away.

You used a sharpening block with various sizes of grooves representing the gauges of needles. The next step was to drag the needle at a 45° angle through the grooves to sharpen it. Then you wiped the needle across a cotton ball to make sure there were no barbs, which obviously would cause a little more pain during an injection. The last step was to place the rack into the autoclave.

The syringes were glass. Both parts, the plunger (that pushes the medication) and the barrel (which held the solution to be injected), were labeled with a corresponding number. We had to match the numbers when assembling the syringe. If the numbers didn't match, the syringe would not function properly. (When you tried to inject the medication, it would squirt out the other end, adding yet another cleanup task.) Once assembled, everything went into the autoclave to be sterilized.

Don't Wind the Thread Too Tight

Sutures used for repairing lacerations in the ER came in a variety of strengths and materials. Some would be absorbed and did not need removal, while others needed to be removed when the wound healed.

Nylon sutures were common, which varied from very fine to a little heavier. Silk sutures were also available. Dr. Mario del Rio, our full-time emergency room physician, preferred 3-0 silk, a rather thick thread for any type of suturing regardless of where the laceration was on the body. I'm guessing it was easier for him to see and tie a strong knot.

Dr. del Rio immigrated from Cuba when he was a little boy. It always puzzled me why he mostly mumbled and pointed. He actually spoke English but was not conversationally understandable. About everybody working in the ER had worked with him for so long that they knew what he wanted. His treatment plan rarely changed.

None of our suture material came prepackaged or labeled so that we could just open a sterile set of sutures and drop it on a tray, ready to use, with the needle attached. We were not so lucky. The sutures came on a spool; we had to cut them into 12-inch or 18-inch lengths to wind around small pieces of cardboard squares with a cut corner. The thread was started in the slit and wound top to bottom, then side to side with the end piece again placed in the slit to fasten the thread to the cardboard.

We need to take care not to wind the threads too tight, because during the autoclave process, they might shrink a little and would be challenging to unwind. After the winding was done, we placed the thread in a marked jar according to size before autoclaving. We retrieved the thread from the jar as needed. That was our golden rule: "Don't wind the thread too tight and don't mix up the sizes." More lessons to learn.

No, You Cannot Autoclave Thermometers!

On one of our busier days, Ms. Aspen requested assistance from another Candy Striper. I was less than thrilled because now this individual was cutting into my territory. But we were busy, and I wanted to help with the patients. Virginia was one year younger than me, 2 inches shorter, and quite a few points lower than the average IQ. I was thrilled to give Virginia her directions on what to do and how to do it.

Wanting to be helpful, Virginia put all the soaked and cleaned thermometers in one of our metal containers, closed the lid, and placed them in the autoclave. The thermometers exploded. Thank God we had a lid on the container, or we would be cleaning up a bigger mess inside the autoclave. Talk about a mercury hazmat situation! I hoped we had more thermometers in the hospital because we sure went through this batch quickly.

There were always more jobs. One of our other tasks in Central Supply was to make a variety of trays for procedures such as for catheterization, tracheostomy, suturing, irrigation, and so on. We had a card that identified the contents of each tray. Once assembled, the trays were wrapped in autoclavable paper and marked and dated.

I was so glad when years later, somebody finally invented disposable products, including needles, syringes, and a variety of trays. This makes nursing a lot easier than spending time assembling supplies. Although, I can't complain because many years ago nurses also washed the floors. So, I guess putting supplies together wasn't such a big deal. When disposables became available, some of the bean counters, better known as the Finance Department, thought it was cheaper to assemble our own trays rather than purchasing disposables. However, there was little consideration given to the amount of nursing time spent in nonpatient activities rather than being at the bedside. Listening to our patients and providing care was just as important as assembling tools for the trade, more critical. Unfortunately, that problem of devaluing nursing time still exists in today's world.

Our Community Emergency Room

The emergency room portion of my experience was fascinating. The ER patients were intriguing. I saw everything from lumps and bumps to sore throats, common colds, broken arms and legs, heart attacks, and car accidents. It was a moderately busy emergency room considering the size of the community.

We weren't staffed by an agency providing physicians trained in emergency medicine. We had Dr. Mario del Rio during the day shift, who did more pointing than speaking. In the evenings and on weekends, our emergency room was staffed with residents moonlighting from a variety of specialties and hospitals. Some of them were good and some seemed to be bothered by the patient showing up in the ER at 2 AM with a blister. This was not exactly an emergency but nonetheless annoying to both the doctor and the staff. I often had to remind myself that an emergency is defined as what the patient thinks is an emergency, and it is not always going to be life-threatening, unless you have the urge to kill them.

Every hospital emergency room has its share of frequent flyers. These are individuals who regularly show up on the doorstep of the emergency department, usually with minor complaints. We all know it's hard to get a doctor's appointment when you feel like hell, so rather than wait, some go to the emergency room. Sometimes these frequent visits are necessary for chronic conditions such as uncontrolled diabetes, recurrent chest pains, hypertensive crisis, or chronic respiratory problems. Most of the time, they usually can wait till you can get into your private family physician's office. But I remember some people define emergencies differently and think everything is an emergency.

One of our frequent flyers on the coldest day in October was brought into the ER by the Police Department. Someone found her lying in the bushes with just a sweater on and one shoe missing. No one knew how long she had been exposed to the elements. Mary was known for her drinking habits, which were not difficult to acquire since our town had a bar on every corner. In her younger days, Mary was quite pretty and enjoyed entertaining the blue-collar men in the community.

When she presented to the emergency room, Mary was not responding and was cold to the touch. Dr. del Rio took one look at her, waved his hand, and said, "She's dead. Put her in the morgue". The nurse and I couldn't feel a pulse either, so we put a sheet over Mary and placed her in the morgue adjacent to the emergency room.

Later that evening, Richard, our maintenance guy and general handyman, got the keys to the morgue to mop the floors. This was one of his less favorite duties since he was terrified of dead people. We often tried to lessen his anxiety by telling him the dead can't hurt him. He still had his doubts. When he opened the door, he found Mary sitting on the cart wrapped with a sheet yelling, "It's so damn cold in here; it's so cold in here." Richard didn't say anything to anybody, he just put down his mop, and walked away. We never saw him again. I often wondered what happened to him. Maybe we should have taken a closer look at Mary when she arrived. While she survived to drink again and continued to be one of our better-known frequent flyers, the takeaway lesson was you can't assume people are dead just because they're cold, don't move, don't talk, and don't have a pulse! They may be just comfortably sleeping in a deep alcohol-induced coma.

When things were quiet in the emergency room, we cleaned. We washed wheelchairs, wheels on the carts, and shelves. Also, we threw out expired medications. There's nothing like having everything you need when you need it. After all, it needed to function as an emergency room. Nobody enjoyed doing spring cleaning on a regular basis, however, Ms. Aspen was a stickler on order and organization. She would've made a great Marine drill sergeant.

I occasionally went upstairs to the nursing units to visit the patients admitted from our emergency room. Patients stayed a lot longer than one day. Doctors discharged them after they felt better or were on their way to recovery. (Today the average length of stay is maybe one-two days if they're lucky. There's a lot of literature to show that some patients recuperate better in their own home, and there is just as much literature to support that a premature discharge leads to readmission, usually in a worse condition.)

I was always impressed by how busy everybody looked and how comfortable the patients were on the nursing units. Activities were quite different on the units than they were in the ER.

Nurses' Aide Role

I soon became more interested in the hands-on aspect of nursing care, so I became a nurses' aide, trading in my red and white Candy Striper uniform for a blue striped pinafore. As a result of my on-the-job training, I was already reasonably familiar with the duties of nurses' aides. I enjoyed taking care of the patients when I worked the afternoon shift. At that time, our activity centered around getting the patients ready for the night.

We bathed patients if needed and changed pillow cases and draw sheets. Everybody got a back rub. This activity relaxed the patients and helped them sleep without the aid of medication. Patients were comfortable and ready for a quiet night. Often in today's world, it seems that bedtime care consists of answering the call light if it goes off, changing the garbage bag, and delivering fresh water to the patient's bedside. Now, sadly back rubs seem to be a thing of the past.

Food service was also a little different. A cart came come up from the kitchen with what looked like tubs of potatoes, vegetables, and the meat of the day. We put the food on warm plates in the hallway and delivered it directly to the patient.

Unfortunately, as a patient, you only had two choices: take it or leave it. Unless you were on a special diet, everybody got the same food. If you were on a special diet, your tray would be brought up from the kitchen and served immediately. The overbed tray was always clean and ready for the meal. This type of food service probably wouldn't be practical or even possible on a much larger scale. Patients knew when breakfast, lunch, and dinner was served, and they knew the food would be hot and good. There were very few complaints.

In our hospital, male and female patients were on separate floors, perhaps because it was a Catholic hospital. Orderlies (the male version of a nurse's aide) and even a male nurse staffed the first floor for male patients. The second floor had female patients and a small pediatric unit. The third floor consisted of the operating rooms, the recovery room, and more female patient beds. Female patients were cared for by female nurses' aides and female nurses. The hospital was not huge nor was it a part of a healthcare conglomerate. Most of the staff worked and lived in the community and usually walked to work.

As a Catholic hospital, we often had an occasional nun or priest as a patient. One such patient was Sr. Mary Constance. Sister had a private room and was more of a resident than a patient even though she had multiple health problems. She had her assigned aide who took excellent care of her. Sr. Constance was disabled with arthritis and could not walk; she could not do much of anything for herself. When her regular aide, Cindy, went on vacation, the nurse manager asked me to take over on the 3 to 11 shift to care for Sr. Constance as her private nurses' aide. Initially, I welcomed the opportunity, but I was soon a little intimidated by Sister who was an extremely demanding individual. Everything was done a certain way and at a specific time with no exceptions. Although she had never been in her bathroom, she could tell you exactly what was on every shelf, where it was located, and how to use it. I needed to irrigate and rebandage multiple pressure injury wounds every evening. Although the process was unimaginably painful, she never complained.

Once the dressings were completed, the next step was to get Sister ready for her 8 PM visit by the Chaplain. That meant making the room perfectly clean and ensuring her veil was straight. Believe me, Sister knew when that veil was not straight even though she couldn't see it or feel with her crippled fingers. The veil application was a challenge for me since it was held in place with several straight pins, and I was terrified of sticking Sister Constance in the head. She was quick to give clear and careful step-by-step instructions. I followed the instructions carefully and we both survived.

Sr. Constance was a challenge but a true inspiration. Despite her adversity and pain, she did what she could and prayed for everybody. I visited her frequently when I was in nursing school to see how she was doing and to tell her of my adventures as a student nurse. As I entered my senior year, the staff told me Sr. Constance was in a coma and was at the end of her life.

Cindy told me that during her lucid moments, Sister said she wanted me to visit. So, I came immediately. Sister Constance was sleeping, or at least appeared to be. When she heard my voice, she opened her eyes and told me that I was going to be a good nurse (even though it had been many years since I cared for her.) We talked a little about school, and shortly after that visit, she passed away in her sleep.

I have fond memories of another patient, our hospital Chaplain, Father Mike. Father Mike developed pneumonia and was quarantined in his room. One of the nuns wanted to bring Father Mike a mustard plaster for his chest and asked me to go with her since she did not feel comfortable being in his room by herself. Truthfully, neither did I. He was drop-dead gorgeous, 6-foot-tall, had piercing blue eyes, blonde wavy hair, and a striking resemblance to Zac Efron. Wow, I didn't mind that visit at all. Now there's a patient I would've wanted to take care of and nurse back to health. He soon recovered and was back to work, saving souls and making hearts beat faster.

TAKING THE NEXT STEPS

I soon advanced to unit secretary. The challenging experience of deciphering doctors' handwriting was helpful when I became a nurse. I could almost second-guess what it was and what they wanted, no matter who the physician was. (Now, with electronic medical records, it makes it so much easier for a physician to order the correct medication since drop-down boxes have the correct spelling.) I often thought physicians wrote the way they did because they forgot how to spell due to the need to quickly take notes in medical school. Many doctors would not have graduated if they had to pass a legible handwriting test. Looking at some of the signatures, we couldn't even tell if they were doctors or just had a twitch in their hand.

I wrote a poem about this:

> *"The doctor is a worthy gent;*
> *The patients claim he's heaven sent.*
> *The man is knowing, erudite;*
> *But, holy cats! He just can't write.*
> *The surgeon's hands are deft and skilled;*
> *The surgeon's head is know-how filled.*
> *Yet why, since he's so doggone bright,*
> *Cannot the surgeon learn to write?*
> *Dear sons of old Hippocrates,*
> *Pray hear a troubled nurse's plea:*
> *Remember that the girls in white*
> *Have got to read the stuff you write!*
> *Your physicals and histories,*
> *Like Dead Sea Scrolls, are mysteries.*
> *Your order sheets, make nurses squint*

So please, dear Sirs, write right, or print!"

This may not be the best poem ever written. I just had to write it at the time, considering my age and some frustration being the unit secretary having to decipher all this. When I shared my poem, the responses from some of the physicians were interesting. Some understood the message but continued to write like they had a gun in their ribs. For me, it was a great learning experience because, as a nurse, I think I could decipher anybody's writing and probably still can to this day. The next step was to select my school of nursing, applying, get accepted, and get started on my career.

CHAPTER THREE

NURSING EDUCATION THEN AND NOW

*"In nursing school, it doesn't matter
if you make the grade when you
don't understand the concepts!"*

— Anonymous

CHOOSING THE RIGHT SCHOOL

How TO CHOOSE the right nursing school for me? The National League for Nursing published a resource guide that identified all the schools of nursing in the greater Detroit, Michigan metropolitan area. Criteria for admission, as well as program descriptions, were available for anyone interested in finding a school of nursing. I was surprised to find out that just about every hospital had its school of nursing, its nursing pin, and distinct nursing philosophy. The hospitals developed diploma nursing programs that also reflected their values and beliefs. Tuition was generally reasonable since the student nurses provided most of the nursing care on the afternoon and midnight shifts. The students were supervised, often by nurses only a few years older than them. A lot of the decision-making reflected the blind leading the blind.

After looking at the information on schools, I again turned to Elaine for some advice. Elaine was a graduate of Saint Joseph Mercy Hospital School of Nursing, a diploma program, which was administered by the Religious Sisters of Mercy. They also governed Mercy College of Detroit, founded in 1941. In 1990, Mercy College of Detroit merged with University of Detroit, founded by the Jesuits in 1877, and renamed University of Detroit Mercy.

Elaine suggested I pursue a bachelor's degree in nursing (BSN) and attend Mercy College. If in the future I wanted to use my degree for a management position, I would have an advantage.

I took Elaine's advice and applied to both Mercy College of Detroit and the University of Michigan. I was accepted at both schools, but I chose Mercy College since it was closer to home, and I could commute to classes. There were times I regretted not going to the big university campus in Ann Arbor and experiencing that college "away from home" spirit. I was serious about my education, so I soon got over it. I was fortunate to obtain a scholarship for 3 of the 4 years I attended school.

How to Survive the Right School

Every school had strict rules and regulations. That's true of any educational program or job. So, I followed the rules *most of the time*. The diploma schools of nursing provided dorms or residences for their students during their enrollment in the program. College students stayed either in the dorm or commuted. There were rules and regulations in the dorm that also had to be followed, if there was to be any order anywhere and to provide students actual quiet time in which to study.

One of the rules at Mercy College was that student nurses could not date the interns. Why not? I suppose it would take us away from our concentration on our studies. My girlfriend Linda and I decided to test the waters since we met two interns who were handsome and interested in dating us. We went on a few dates; it was exciting to hear the other students talk about: "I wonder who the nursing students are who were dating the interns." They never suspected Linda or I, so we had fun with our little secret. The romance was exciting while it lasted.

The curriculum of the first year of school had a lot of science, English, and general college-level liberal arts classes. Anatomy and physiology, biochemistry, and other typical science classes required in most of the nursing programs at that time. I cut open frogs and cats, played with Bunsen burners, and tried not to burn the labs down. I was fascinated with the science classes and the experiments. My instructors were far more interested in the experiment outcomes, which didn't always come out as planned. That's what school is all about, learning from your mistakes. I learned a lot.

My Brains Are Not Attached to My Nursing Cap

Sometime between the first and second year my instructors noticed I had experience with the American Red Cross as a volunteer and as a fantastic Candy Striper. The Rev. Victoria Meadows approached me, after speaking with the Dean, to teach a Home Nursing Class for the Nurses Guild in her church. The American Red Cross sponsored these programs as well as Basic First Aid classes. Since nursing was my passion, I was honored for the invitation. The classes were simple. I taught the ladies how to read a thermometer, which wasn't always easy with bifocals and those itty-bitty little numbers with mercury in between.

I also taught them the difference between a rectal and an oral thermometer. In this digital age, I don't think there are too many glass thermometers left in use. I taught how to feed the patient without choking him. My students learned how to tie a knotted rope to the end of the bed so the patient could grab the rope by the knots and pull himself up to a sitting position. They learned how to fold a newspaper to make a disposable bag for tissues, reposition patients using several pillows, and make a wedge out of a paper box.

My Nursing Guild ladies wore white uniforms at the services. Some purchased nursing caps at the local uniform store and they had their fancy lace breast pocket handkerchiefs in case someone fainted and needed to be fanned. They were a dedicated group; I loved teaching this class and sharing my passion. We laughed a lot, and I learned as much from them as they did from me.

The class took place before our capping ceremony. I approached the Dean to see if I could get my nursing cap early so, I would look more like a nurse teaching the class. Her answer was "no". She informed me it would be far more meaningful when I received my nursing cap with the entire class. She then reminded me that my brains are not attached to my cap. I was perfectly capable of teaching what I needed to teach without my cap.

She was right. My ladies accepted me as I was and shared my enthusiasm for helping those in need. As our capping ceremony approached, I was excited to finally look like a nurse. As far as functioning as a nurse, I had a long way to go. However, the image was important to my fellow classmates and me. Once I received my cap, my clinical rotations would start. I soon learned how to think like a nurse, not just look like one. I was excited and terrified at the same time.

ON TO MY CLINICAL ROTATIONS

The class was divided into smaller groups. My clinical group was assigned to Mount St. Helen Hospital, six floors with approximately 700 patient beds. At my preclinical conference, I met my clinical instructor, Ms. Barbara Singular. She defined her expectations. She smiled a lot, which made me wonder what she knew that I didn't know that made her so happy. Maybe she just liked teaching.

Ms. Singular told us to come directly to the conference room on our clinical rotation days and not to stop along the way. As luck would have it, I was walking down the hall when one of the doctors stuck his head out of the room and said, "Nurse, would you help me?" I remember my instructor's words and said to him, " Oh, I'm not a nurse." He looked at me and said, "You look like a nurse; you're dressed like a nurse, and it's way too early for Halloween. All I want you to do is to hold this dressing so I can tape it in place". I could do that, so I did. Wouldn't you know it, the first person I saw as I was walking out of the patient's room with him was my instructor. Oops, I was busted! She just looked at me and didn't say anything. You know that kind of look; we've all seen it. The doctor was kind enough to explain. Thank you, Doctor!

Dressing for our clinical destination was different than it is today. I didn't wear scrubs; I wore a white uniform, and the emphasis was on the word *white*. I was not allowed to wear my uniform to and from the hospital. I brought my uniform and changed at the hospital. Heaven forbid I should bring in germs from the outside to the patient's bedside. I often wondered if anyone considered that doctors wore the same outfit from room to room. Visitors sat on the patient's bed, leaving some germs behind, I'm sure. I wasn't able to argue with the concept.

One traumatic day I forgot my white stockings. Oh no, now what? There was no place to get a pair, and I didn't have the time anyway. The only thing I could think of was to grab the white shoe polish and rub it on my legs. I prayed that nothing spilled on them to make my nylons disappear. I stayed very low on my instructor's radar that day and, since I'm as pale as a ghost, it worked.

A Different Use for Urinals and Other Embarrassing Moments

It did not sound complicated when a patient's family brought flowers in and asked me to put them in the vase. I headed for clean utility room to look for a vase. I didn't find any glass vases, but there was a whole bunch of narrow metal vases with handles. So, I put the flowers in a metal vase and proceeded to march down the hall holding the handle like a bride. My instructor came running after me yelling, "That's not a vase; that's not a vase." It looked like a vase to me, and I thought it was a nifty idea putting on handles. She educated me on the use of urinals. Oops! Remember, my background was working with female patients; I had no idea what a urinal was. I do now.

That was not my only embarrassing encounter that week. It seemed that the interns and residents had a lot of fun teasing the student nurses. I was trying to observe a bedside procedure, when the resident on the case sent me, STAT, to central supply (CSR) for a fallopian tube. I didn't give any thought to the order; I just went immediately to CSR on the 6th floor. The department manager, who was a rather cranky/crabby older individual, didn't particularly like students.

When I asked for a fallopian tube, she looked at me and asked, "Did you flunk anatomy?" "No, I was pretty good at anatomy." "Then what do you think a fallopian tube is?" I immediately wanted to slither out of her presence. However, I politely apologized for disturbing her; and yes, I do know what a fallopian tube is. I learned a valuable lesson: put your brain in gear before your body in motion. Had I stopped to think about what the resident was asking for, I would have avoided placing myself in that embarrassing situation. My next stop would have been to scold the resident. I wanted to give him a piece of my mind but decided to wait for a better opportunity.

I wasn't the only student nurse having issues with time management and organization. I ran into one of my high school classmates, Karen, who was attending Rivard Hospital School of Nursing. Rivard Hospital was built during the Civil War and still had many eight-bed wards. She told me that she and another classmate were assigned to one of the eight-bed wards. Their job was to do the baths, make sure the beds were clean, nightstands straightened out, and patients happy. This sounded reasonable and not too far-fetched from my clinical duties.

As she explained, Karen was running late one day, so she decided to grab a big pan of water and collect all the dentures in one pan and clean them at one time rather than individually. She cleaned all the dentures in a hurry, but when it came time to return them to the owner, that was a big problem. She first showed them to the patients in hopes they could recognize their own dentures. That worked for just a few. For the rest, Karen had no recourse other than to have the patients try on the denture, and if it fit, they owned it. Kudos for thinking out of the box. However, sometimes you just must think a plan through before you execute it. That was a good lesson for me.

BEDPAN ALLEY

Anyone who has worked in health care knows the importance and usefulness of a bedpan. We all must use them at some point when you can't get out of bed and walk to the bathroom. Little has changed over the years except for the fact that today's bedpans are plastic, warmer, and come in a variety of sizes and shapes. Many years ago, bedpans were metal, cold, and one-size-fits-all.

The postoperative floors, especially orthopedics, were affectionately referred to as "bedpan alley." Nobody got out of bed. If you are walking around, you don't need to be in a hospital. A thoughtful nurse who had time would run warm water in the pan to warm it up, then sliding it under the patient. This was not always possible, but it was a good idea, along with powdering the edge to facilitate placement and removal.

Modern hospitals have a flushable unit attached directly to the toilet in the patient's room. During my school days, no such thing existed. We had covers that looked like part of a pillowcase into which you slid the bedpan and carefully proceeded to the dirty utility room where you disposed of the contents. Since the bedpans were metal, there was a wall unit hopper that provided a cleaning action and sterilized the metal bedpan. The operation was simple. You carefully opened the hopper door (it opened like an oven door), placed the bedpan into the frame, then carefully closed and secured the hopper door. Once you were sure that the hopper door was locked, you pushed the button that delivered a spray of steam, enough to empty the contents of the bedpan and sterilize it. One of the first things I learned about the hopper was to stay clear of that door, just in case it wasn't latched properly. I will let your imagination go to what could happen.

On one of my hectic clinical days, I had a patient who frequently urinated into the bedpan. As I was ready to leave for a post clinical conference, she needed the bedpan again. Okay, that's what I'm here for, to take care of the patient. I didn't want to be late for the conference. I took the rather full bedpan, covered it, and ran out of the room just in time to run into the Chief of Medicine and deposit the contents of that bedpan onto his shirt and tie. He didn't say anything; he didn't have to. I had a towel slung over my shoulder, so I started wiping him up. I apologize profusely as I was rubbing the urine into his shirt. The only comment he made was, "Don't rub it in."

I was horrified! I thought my nursing career was going to end right there. I had to explain to my clinical instructor why I was late. I told her what happened in hopes of getting some sympathy. She explained to me she knew the physician and his personality. She was amazed that he didn't remove my head from my shoulders. He was rather understanding of the circumstances and apparently, this wasn't his first christening by a student. Another important lesson learned: haste makes waste.

MOMS AND BABIES

My first day in the obstetrics clinical rotation was scheduled the day before we had any lecture material. I was kind of clueless. My classmate Marilyn and I were assigned to the bedside of a patient in active labor. The doctor came in to examine the patient and told us, "Just watch her, when she starts to crown, let me know."

We read the chapter ahead of time; we were pretty sure we thought what crowning meant. We decided to wait until the next contraction to see what happened. When we spotted the baby's head, we both left to get the doctor. Just then, our instructor, Ms. Debbie Butler, walked in and wanted to know who was watching the patient. I explained that Marilyn and I were watching the patient and left to get the doctor, per his request. She patiently explained that obviously, we weren't the brightest bulbs in the chandelier because we abandoned the patient. Marilyn and I heard a list of what-ifs and were convinced we had a lot to learn in obstetrics. Our mom went on to safely deliver her little boy.

Delivery practices have also changed over the years. Fathers were not allowed in the delivery room. They paced in the waiting area until the announcement of their new addition to the family. Fathers were often not allowed to even touch the newborn for fear of giving the baby germs.

Modern obstetric (OB) practices allow fathers to be at the bedside throughout the labor, often involved in coaching the mom, and to cut the cord after delivery. Midwives and birthing coaches (doulas) assist mom during labor and delivery, frequently in the home rather than a hospital. Babies are born in warm tubs of water, representing their uterine environment. Nurses don't shave mothers for delivery, nor are they always given an enema.

During my OB rotation, it was customary practice to shave the perineum so the mother's pubic hair would not interfere or possibly cause an infection during delivery. I quickly learned that babies have no sense of timing and didn't always want to wait for me to get my act together. One such incident occurred when the mother was already in the delivery room, and I had to shave the perineum. My instructor told me to hurry, so I did. I just shaved right straight down the middle; as she pushed, I gave the baby its first haircut. I was horrified! I thought the baby's brains would fall out or something. The obstetrician thought it was funny. My instructor assured me that the brains were well protected. She then asked what time the baby was born, since I was supposed to track that in the medical record. I had no idea. I didn't look at the clock; I was too busy worrying about what I just did. The obstetrician was kind enough to give us the time of birth so we can officially put it on the birth certificate—what a relief. I learned a lot that day, mostly to pay attention to what I was doing and to speed it up.

Mysteries of the Human Mind

My psychiatric nursing rotation was different from anything I did in the adult medical-surgical areas.

Some of the patients had chronic medical conditions but had mental health issues that superseded whatever else may have been a comorbidity.

Eastville State Hospital was a multi-building campus that provided housing for male, female, and adolescent mental health patients. My class was assigned to building L, which housed female patients. This was a locked unit. I was issued a key and told to keep it out of sight and make sure the door was always locked after I entered, and when I left. No problem there, I didn't want anybody to leave who shouldn't.

One clinical day I had the key pinned to the inside seam of my jumper. I was in a hurry to get out and lock the door as a patient was approaching. The key was in the door, and I slammed it, managing to tear the front of my jumper and show my slip. At least it was clean and pretty, but a bit embarrassing. Safety was always a concern, and safety pins were a blessing.

I was warned not to be alone in the bathroom or shower areas with a patient. On one occasion, I was washing a patient's hair in the sink. She was getting very agitated because it took me so long to rinse. Her head didn't exactly fit under the faucet, and she had long hair. I turned around and noticed the patient and I were the only individuals in the room. I was a little nervous until one of the attendants came in looking for my patient. I was happy to turn her over to someone else.

It was interesting to try to talk to the patients to gain their trust so they would speak openly and speak to me. When my patient sat quietly, I sat quietly, allowing her to make the first move towards the conversation. That didn't seem to work because another patient approached us and asked if I was a new patient. At that point, I felt like I could have been.

My clinical group had a field trip to Calmwood, a private mental health facility. This was very different from the state-owned facility. The grounds were well landscaped, the building was well equipped and staffed. Our instructor, Ms. Rosie Blue, gave us specific instructions to wait in the lobby for her because she was running a little late. By now, I got the message to follow instructions. My class and I waited in the lobby, and soon, a gentleman showed up wearing a lab coat and asked if we were the students for the tour. I informed him that we were waiting for our instructor. He told us that we needed to start the tour immediately if we were going to finish, adding that our instructor has been there many times and was aware of how long it takes for the tour.

So, my classmates and I followed him like lemmings. As we went from ward to ward, he identified some of the mental health issues with the patients. He pointed out one lady who was crying in the corner and stated, "She thinks she's Mary Magdalene. She keeps crying; and the gentleman seated on the couch, he thinks he's St. Peter and of course is very dedicated to studying his books and the Bible." Moving on to another ward, several patients were playing cards. Our guide identified them as part of the 12 apostles. Now I was getting a little suspicious, so I asked, "Excuse me, I didn't catch your name." He said, "Oh, I'm sorry I didn't introduce myself. I'm Jesus Christ".

An attendant soon showed up looking for our tour guide. Just about the same time, our instructor came storming down the hallway. I knew I was in trouble along with my classmates. She reminded us that mental health patients can be extremely unpredictable, and we could've been in grave danger. Ms. Blue revealed that many years ago, she worked in a hospital school of nursing, where seven students were killed by a psychiatric patient who managed to get into their dorm room. One student hid under the bed and escaped to reveal the details of that horrible scene. Another important lesson learned: things aren't always what they seem.

SMALL PATIENTS WITH BIG PROBLEMS

Our pediatric clinical rotation was in Children's Hospital, which was built around the turn-of-the-century. There are multiple sixand eightbed wards to accommodate children of different ages and stages of development. There were isolation rooms, even an isolation diarrhea ward accommodating 4 to 5 cribs. I had a lot to learn to switch to a pediatric population after working with adults. Our lectures covered many syndromes and diseases affecting children. We learned about growth and development at different stages of life and what was normal and abnormal.

During our clinical rotations, we were assigned by twos to the various wards. We worked as a team to assess the patients, keep them comfortable, entertained, and, most important, quiet. No one likes to see children in pain. It was hard for children to understand why specific procedures or examinations had to be done to help them get better. It was not always easy to explain to the child or to the parent who was ever vigilant.

My instructor assigned me to an eight-month-old baby with cystic fibrosis. It is difficult for children with this disease to clear their lungs of fluid. One of the exercises was to place the baby on your lap and gently thump (percuss) on the back to loosen secretions. I was waiting for the mother to arrive, so I could demonstrate this procedure for her to continue when the child was discharged. The mom walked in, just as I was getting started and was upset that I was beating up her baby. I quickly explained to her that I was not beating up her baby but was trying to loosen secretions to help the baby breathe easier. Mom calmed down after she saw the baby's breathing was somewhat relieved. I showed her how to do the exercise. It was a brief scary moment since mom was quite upset.

As I progressed with my training, my instructor assigned me to the treatment room to assist with holding the child for a procedure or treatment. They wiggle and occasionally pee on you. Therefore, you plan on how you can safely restrain the child and make sure the diaper is fastened well. Sometimes singing to the children or rocking them before the procedure helped to calm them down.

Speaking of diapers, I was also assigned to the diarrhea isolation ward. This was no fun; the children needed many diaper changes. I quickly learned how to keep the diapers from falling off. One of my patients was an 18-month-old with flaming red curly hair. As I just finished removing his diaper and washing him, one of the residents came in and picked him up. I strongly suggested putting him down and let me put on another diaper. Too late – another bout of diarrhea rolled down the resident's lab coat, pants, and shoes. My reflexes were better; I moved out of the way. I offered to help him clean up, but he declined and slunk off the ward.

An assignment to the orthopedic children's ward didn't go much better. Since they weren't physically sick, just in plaster, it was a more significant challenge to keep them entertained and out of mischief. The frames on the bed that suspended the traction usually looked like little cages, which was appropriate in many instances. On one such occasion, my instructor walked into the room just as I was stopping my patient from swinging from the overhead traction bar belonging to his roommate. I managed to tackle him and return him to his bed because I promised to read him a story if he behaved. My instructor was not exactly impressed with my bedside manner, but it worked. I survived pediatrics and knew this was not my favorite rotation. Kids get sick fast, but they also get well quickly, which is an advantage.

More Opportunities for Learning

During my senior year, I was hired as a student nurse in the Emergency Room at Blessed Redeemer Hospital. Blessed Redeemer was a busy community hospital that served many small industries. We were busy with a variety of industrial-type accidents, including lacerations, fractures, and traumatic amputations of fingers and toes.

Every Saturday, the Emergency Department had an Orthopedic Clinic for follow-up since most of our industrial accidents were orthopedic related. The clinic was run by two orthopedic physicians who were brothers, Dr. Samuel Handy and Dr. John Handy. Both were dedicated to orthopedics with Dr. Samuel Handy doing additional research through the Veterans Administration with soldiers returning from duty with amputations. They loved to teach, and that strengthened my interest in orthopedics.

One of my coworkers, Ronald Conklin, also shared my interest in orthopedics, particularly foot injuries. He was fascinated with the concept of biomechanics related to the foot since he was studying engineering at the time. Ron went on to study Podiatric Medicine. Apparently, that wasn't the only thing he was fascinated with since he became the love of my life and my husband shortly after graduation.

STUDENT NURSE OF THE YEAR... BASKING IN THE GLORY!

Throughout my nursing education, I was always involved with the National Student Nursing Association on campus. The organization's mission was to bring together and mentor students preparing for initial licensure as registered nurses. It also conveyed the standards and ethics of the nursing profession. Through its meetings and conferences, students developed skills they would need as responsible and accountable members of the nursing profession. I was a delegate to the national convention held in Michigan in my senior year.

Shortly before the conference, I was approached by the Dean to answer a few questions at the request of the National Student Nursing Association. I didn't want to be bothered because I was busy studying. Also, I had the added responsibilities of being a delegate to the convention. But, when the Dean asks you to do something, you do it. So, I did.

Four essay type questions dealt with how you, as a student, viewed the future of nursing as a profession. That didn't sound too difficult. I had opinions, and I had no problem expressing them. I wasn't too sure why I was being asked these questions; I answered to the best of my ability. When I attended the convention, I met one of my high school classmates, Carol Knapp, who was attending another college of nursing and was also a delegate. We sat next to each other and reminisced a lot about the good old days in high school.

As the program progressed, the president of the National Student Nursing Association announced that the decision was made regarding the Student Nurse of The Year for the State of Michigan. Rather than announcing the name of the recipient, she started reading the responses to the essay questions. I heard the first essay response; it sounded good. Then she read the second essay response. Now that was starting to sound familiar. Moving on to the third essay response, I knew that was mine. I excitedly poked Carol and told her, "That was me, that was me!" She slowly looked at me and said "Yeah, sure".

Then the moment of truth: the fourth essay response was read. I was officially named Michigan's Student Nurse of the Year. I was so excited. I turned around, and I saw the Dean and a lot of faculty members in attendance. The master of ceremonies asked me to come on stage and make some remarks. I think for the first time in my life, I was speechless. I managed to say a few words (I can't remember what they were) but the audience clapped. I sat down before I said something stupid. What an exciting day. The next step was the big one: graduation and State Boards.

CHAPTER FOUR

GRADUATION AND STATE BOARDS

*"Nursing school is a lot like giving birth…
once it's over, you tend to forget just
how painful the process really was."*

— Anonymous

GRADUATION DAY FINALLY came. Along with my classmates, we celebrated our successes and looked forward to the future. The future meant Michigan State Board of Nursing exam for licensure. Our journey was just beginning, although when we started it, it seemed like we would never finish. Suddenly the end was here. Now the buck stops with me. Did I learn enough? Will I remember when the times comes? Only time will tell.

I Look Like a Nurse, I'm Scared

After graduation on May 10, 1969, my status at Blessed Redeemer Hospital changed from student nurse in the Emergency Room to Graduate Nurse on a surgical unit. I was excited to learn as much as I could, but it was very different from the emergency room. Prioritization and organization were critical factors for survival. I had to get better at both. I spent a lot of time running back and forth either to the patient's room or to the utility room to get something I forgot. My grandmother always said, "If your brain is not in gear, your legs will be in motion." I never quite understood what that meant until I became a nurse.

What Could They Possibly Ask on the State Board RN Licensing Exam?

The next venture was State Board Exams. Some of us had thought that if you didn't learn it by now, you're not going to learn it by cramming those couple months before the exam. I graduated in May, and the State Boards were scheduled in July and October in Lansing, Michigan, our state capital. I had to travel to Lansing to take the exam, approximately 95 miles from home. Unlike today's state board exams, which are offered in numerous places on computers, mine was a paper and pencil exam. I shared an auditorium like space with some 200 students, with proctors walking up and down the aisles, making sure nobody was cheating.

The exams were divided into adult med/surg, obstetrics, psychiatry, and pediatrics. There were some test questions added for future exams depending on the results. The questions were all multiple choice, or multiple guess, and presented as a scenario followed by questions. The exams were scheduled for a morning and afternoon session for two days. Unlike today's exam, which has a variety of question formats including multiple-choice, fill in the blanks, choose all that apply, etc., ours was simple, multiple guess only.

GETTING THE RESULTS: I PASSED, I'M OFFICIALLY A REGISTERED NURSE, I THINK!

One of the advantages that I had was that I could work as a graduate nurse before I had the results of my state board exam. This was the same job and almost the equal pay as a registered nurse, but it gave me a little bit more hands-on practical experience that I could gain before I sat for the state boards. When you took your state board exam if you passed, you got a business size letter addressed to you with your name, RN behind it. If you did not pass, you received a bigger envelope with your scores, where you are weak, where you need to improve, and what the process is for reapplying for retaking the exam. It was simply addressed to your first and last name, and sadly no RN behind your name.

The year I graduated, they decided to do away with the business envelope and just send everybody the same envelope with no indication of RN status. So, I was afraid to open it when it arrived because I thought I failed for sure. I couldn't believe I wouldn't pass the state board exam! I got brave and opened the envelope. To my surprise and great relief, I passed. I was so excited: I passed, I passed, I am finally a Registered Nurse (RN). I made it. I couldn't wait to change my graduate nurse status to registered nurse.

Some nurses never bothered to take the exam and become an RN. The pay was about the same; the work was the same; they just had GN behind their name instead of RN. This was common practice for nurses who came from foreign countries where they were recognized for their education and practice as registered nurses but did not wish to take the State Board Exam in Michigan.

Look out Florence Nightingale, here I come! Now onto my first real job as an RN. I learned a lot, and now is my opportunity to prove it.

CHAPTER FIVE

MY FIRST JOB, YES, NOW I AM A NURSE

"Your days can be stressful and exhausting and sometimes thankless. But through long shifts and late nights-the hectic scrum of the emergency room, or in those quiet acts of humanity-you are saving lives, you are offering solace, you're helping to make us a better nation."

—President Barack Obama

ORIENTATION, I HOPE I REMEMBER EVERYTHING

Now THAT I passed my state boards, I continued my work at Blessed Redeemer Hospital as an RN instead of a GN. It was a little scary, but I was ready for it. I left the Emergency Room and moved to a large and busy medical-surgical unit. I worked the afternoon shift, which allowed me to have some freedom with my time management and get better organized without the hassle of all the interruptions during the day shift.

There were a lot of post operative surgical patients coming back to the unit on the afternoon shift, so it was a busy period, and I rapidly learned to prioritize. Postoperative patients needed several assessments:

- was my patient breathing,

- was my patient in pain,

- were the dressings dry and intact, and

- who do I call if I found something unexpected?

I don't care where you went to nursing school, or what degrees you have; you will always prioritize and assess your patient so that your interventions are appropriate.

Before electronic medical records and the ability to copy everything, documentation was color-coded. The day shift wrote in blue or black ink, the afternoon shift documented in green ink, and the night shift documented in red. This made it easy to locate details by the shift. While that sounds a little strange, it was easy to turn to those pages and investigate your patient's condition on the previous shift and the previous day. This was a faster process than the current one using electronic medical records.

The whole purpose of documentation is to communicate effectively. Nurses document what they want the next shift to know, what they did, what they didn't do, and what needs to be followed up. Nursing is a 24/7 profession, and what one shift doesn't finish, the next shift does.

I learned in giving report to the oncoming shift that it was essential to

- identify the patient's emergency contact,

- review and adjust the plan of care, and

- explain what the next nurse could expect from the patient in the next 8 hours or during the next shift.

That sometimes gets missed in an electronic medical record.

Charting on paper involved recording data and noting trends. You had to think before you documented, so the information was coherent, clear, and concise. We charted as we cared for the patient. There were no drop-down boxes. With today's electronic medical records, it is not clear where to document the information if it is not available in the drop-down box. When I documented information, it was current and important, and it wasn't in 16 different areas and 16 different places. It was in the nurses' notes. If anybody wanted to see what kind of day the patient had, it was quite easy to pick up the record and look.

When I started my career as a registered nurse, medical records were not photocopied. As hospital staff recognized the need to share medical records with other providers, it became necessary to make some changes. One of them was to eliminate the color coding for nursing documentation since the copy machine only recognizes black or blue ink. Also, it was critical to document the date and time on every page, so when records were dropped, which they often were, the staff member could reassemble the chart. Otherwise, it was difficult to follow the train of thought in the documentation, who was notified, why, and when. The same holds today for any nurse when it comes to communication and documentation. There are many members on the healthcare team who need to be informed of progress, or lack thereof, concerning the patient's outcome and response to care. The medical record must reflect that communication.

As a new nurse, I discovered I need to give the physician as much information about the patient as possible when I called the physician. This was especially important when speaking with the house physician who worked afternoon and midnight shifts. It was evident to me they were clueless about the patient, so I had to be concise and informative to get the results that I wanted. Heaven forbid you should wake up an attending physician at 2:00 AM to ask for a pain pill or a repeat on pain medication prescribed earlier as a "one time dose".

As a new nurse, I constantly learned lessons. One was to ask for what I needed before the physician went to sleep so I could take care of the sicker patients on the nursing unit. I rapidly learned that if I kept the postoperative patients comfortable with pain medication, both the patients and I would have a better shift. They would be rested, comfortable, and I would not be frantically running around trying to keep everything organized, especially on a busy floor.

The work schedule was crucial. Your work schedule was set in stone. You did not tell your manager that you wanted every Tuesday off because you bowl or that you needed every Friday off before your weekend if you're scheduled to work so that you could party. You were assigned a schedule, and you worked it. There was no question; there was no negotiation. These were your assigned days to come in, and that's what you did. You worked 5 days a week, 8 hours a day. There was no way to determine when your phone rang that the hospital was calling you to ask you to work an extra shift. You could not dodge the call, as is possible now.

We had vacation days and sick time. Some organizations paid in November any time you had accumulated and didn't use from your vacation bank or sick time. That came in handy for Christmas shopping. Other organizations allowed you to bank your vacation days up to a specific limit and take a long vacation if scheduling permitted at some point. This had some drawbacks since individuals who wanted to save up their sick and vacation time showed up for work ill when they should have stayed home.

You Want Me to Work When?

You were occasionally asked to work a double shift due to a colleague's illness. There were days when you barely survived one shift let alone two, but you did what you had to do for the sake of patient care and possibly your career. There were no unions; you followed the rules of the organization, or you moved on to another facility.

Just like today's patient population, some patients were a pleasure to care of, and others were a nightmare. You didn't debate your assignment; you cared for the patients assigned to you. The previous shift made the assignments based on the patients' needs and sometimes knowing the oncoming shift nurses' skill level. If the previous shift liked you, you had a good assignment. If, for whatever reason, they didn't like you, you got the crappiest, worst patients on the floor. That has not changed over the years. We did not have a lot of agency nurses adding to the staff. We had our own staff, and we took care of everything that required attention. After all, it was *our* unit.

Nursing is not an easy profession, either emotionally or physically. You can't help but get attached to your patients. They have needs; sometimes, you are the only one fulfilling those needs. When I had time, I talked to my patients. I visited with their families; I got to know them. Patient stays were a lot longer than they are today, which has become drive through care. They're here today and, if you have two days off, they won't be there when you return. This makes it hard to establish a good nurse-patient rapport. It is also challenging for a good nurse to answer questions, allay some patients' fears, and have an opportunity to teach them about their illness and what the future may hold. Some patients were going home to a nurturing environment, and some were going back to an empty house to take care of themselves.

I often worried about my patients and elicited the help of the Social Services Department to make sure they had a safe discharge plan. In today's healthcare environment, the case manager can take over that role and assist with the resources necessary for the patient to heal and have positive outcomes.

You Never Know What's on Their Mind

Over the years, medications have also changed. Some of the old medications were effective but had side effects, as is true today. We used a lot of Demerol (a pain medication). Demerol had a lot of side effects and is not used as commonly now.

I remember one patient whose Demerol doses almost ended my career. His name was Joe. He worked as an orderly in the Merchant Marine Hospital. The hospital was designed to take care of members of the Merchant Marine who worked the freighters on the Detroit River. Joe was jaundiced and convinced he had cancer. The surgeon who performed surgery determined Joe did *not* have cancer. I talked to Joe a lot to try to convince him that he did not have cancer. I took the pathology report out of a medical record and showed it to Joe. Although it was not common for nurses to show patients parts of their medical records, I felt it was more important for Joe to understand that he was not dying of cancer and would be OK.

One evening on a warm summer's day, the hospital air conditioner wasn't working, and so a lot of the patients opened the windows to get at least a little cool breeze in the evening. (Today it is unusual for hospitals to have windows that open.) I gave Joe his Demerol and again tried to comfort him. I noticed his window was open wide, so I shut it. When I left my shift, Joe jumped out of the window. His room was on the 4th floor. Joe did not die; he fell on a pile of rubble that was the results of some reconstruction at the hospital.

The next day when I came to work, I sat in the cafeteria before my shift to get some coffee and talk to some of the nurses. I heard them asking, "Did you hear about the nurse who gave the patient the wrong medication, and he jumped out the window?" I said, "No, what happened?" The attending physician felt that Demerol caused Joe's psychosis. He gave a verbal order to the head nurse, who often made rounds with physicians, to discontinue the Demerol. She forgot to write it as a verbal order. A 72-hour automatic stop order covered the Demerol by pharmacy, so it was OK for me to give it at 10:00 PM when I did.

I was horrified! I thought, "Oh my God, my career is rapidly going down the toilet!" I could see this as the end of all my hard work. Joe was in a private room and, since I had a good rapport with him, the staff assigned me to do private duty and take care of him for the rest of the shift. Joe had multiple fractures and was in and out of consciousness, but he recovered from his injuries and finally believed he was cancer-free.

The lesson learned was if you're given a verbal order for goodness sake, write it down! Take the time to listen to your patients and do what you can to help them. Looking back on the situation, what I probably should have done was to contact the attending physician and make him more aware of Joe's continued fear of dying of cancer and see if there was anything else I could have done for Joe. Hindsight is always 100%, another lesson learned.

CHAPTER SIX

PUBLIC HEALTH NURSING

"I'm an ex-convict. I have AIDS. I'm a prostitute. I'm poor. I'm old. I'm a lesbian. I aborted my baby. I'm a teenage mom. I'm a victim of rape. I'm a drug addict. I'm alcoholic. I'm a beggar. I have cancer. I have a contagious disease…but the nurse said, 'I'll take care of you.'"

— Anonymous

RON AND I married the August after my graduation. I decided I wanted to work the day shift and spend my evenings with my new husband. The City of Detroit was looking for public health nurses with a bachelor's degree. I was qualified and applied to become a public health nurse.

I started with the Public Health Department City of Detroit NE Health Center. Miss Fitzgibbons was our manager. As a public health nurse for over 30 years, she knew her stuff. She often commented that I was somewhat naïve but would learn if I was interested. Some of the more experienced public health nurses laughed at my comments, and I soon found out that public health nursing was different. Public health nurses did a lot of medical social work by referring people to agencies that could help them. The patients needed jobs and medical attention. The nurses provided more than just hands-on physical nursing.

At first, I thought, "I'm going to forget all my skills. I don't need to give any injections in the home." Therefore, the manager assigned me to an immunization clinic. The health department provided immunizations for children and adults, set up either at a school or at the Health Center. After immunizing over 200 individuals in one day, I decided I was not going to forget my injection skills.

'Don't Get into a Police Car!'

As a public health nurse, I carried a manual which was called our "Bible". It had information on various agencies and procedures that are done at the bedside. I took my black bag loaded with educational material, disinfecting soap, paper towels, and a blood pressure cuff. Based on the assumption that the patient's environment would not be clean, I carried a newspaper to place under my bag. I supplied my own stethoscope and a small pad to keep notes of my visits, which I later transcribed to the patient's medical record stored at the Health Center.

What struck me as peculiar was the first rule in our Bible was, "Do not get into a police car." I thought that was odd. Aren't all police officers willing to help you? Why wouldn't you get into a police car? My coworkers recognized my naivety and reminded me that not all police officers are nice. Some would like to take advantage of pretty young nurses. Really? I never thought that would happen, but apparently, it did, not to me but another nurse.

For my protection, the department was strict about wearing my uniforms and winter coats provided by the public health department. The people in the neighborhood knew I was "the nurse," and I was OK. The manager assigned me to a district that was approximately 5-mile square with an intense patient load. Often I could see several families on the same block. Two smaller cities bordered my district.

There were certain dangerous areas of the City of Detroit that we were not allowed to visit. One of the streets was called Dellmead. Nurses were not allowed to visit on that specific block because it was unsafe.

One day I had a visit scheduled in an apartment building that was on a corner of Oakwood and Dellmead. This was an area where policewomen went by twos, and they were armed. I was wondering if this was a place where I should not be by myself. I decided to be careful and complete the visit. If the individual wasn't home, I would mark the record "not at home" or "not available" and I would try the following day to revisit.

As I entered the apartment building, I followed a trail of blood all the way up to the apartment. I noticed blood smeared on the door. I wondered if there was an injured individual who I could help (as a former ER nurse.) When I heard a lot of noise on the other side of the door, I decided to mark the record as "not at home visit" and check before I tried this address again.

Sometimes common sense takes over no matter how naïve I could be. As I stood there, I fought with my conscience, wondering if I was doing the right thing. Maybe somebody was bleeding, and I could have stopped it. I concluded that I should leave and check on the patient later. I did, and there actually was nobody home at that time. I was relieved and never found out what happened behind that door.

Part of my Health Department duties was to check on the students with health problems. I saw children in school who had chronic diseases, educated the teaching staff, and checked to see how the student was doing in class. One of my schools was Southern High School, with an enrollment of 4000 students. This school only had a part-time school nurse, so the Health Department filled in the gaps. I followed the students of families who were enrolled in our Health Center and any pregnant students.

The gym teacher, Mr. Roberts, was the one assigned to track all these individuals. He supplied me with a student whose job was to retrieve students I needed to see. When I asked him if he had any pregnant students, he laughed. Then he pulled out his stack of index cards that listed 125 pregnant girls currently in school. All of them probably could use attention.

At the time we were meeting, a fight broke out in the gymnasium where one of the girls, who was pregnant, started to miscarry. Her boyfriend found out and stormed into the gym, screaming hysterically, "What did you do to her?" at the gym teacher. I had to deal with a bleeding patient, hysterical boyfriend, and a bunch of screaming kids. Where do I start! Mr. Roberts called for an ambulance (this was before 911 was well-established) to take the student to the hospital. Things eventually settled down through the cool head of the gym teacher, who certainly knew how to handle rowdy teenagers a lot better than I did.

The other school I visited was the Bailey School for Boys. This was part of the city public school system, and it was a school for juvenile delinquents. It was phrased as "students with behavioral issues, general lack of school social skills, and anger management." This school had no more than 200 students. The principal was an ex-marine drill sergeant. When I first walked into his office, he grabbed a student by the collar and slammed him against the wall and shouted, "Behave or else!" I wasn't convinced I wanted to stick around and see what "else" was, but he sure got that kid's attention!

The assistant principal told me, "The principal kind of comes off rough." No kidding! But then he took the kids on camping trips and bought some clothes and things they needed. He served as the father figure for the majority of them. He was quite strict with many rules.

One of the schools' staff asked me to follow up on a student, who was an excellent student but was absent for several days. I visited the home and found deplorable, unsafe conditions. The only light in this upstairs flat was a bare light bulb hanging in the middle of the room between the kitchen and the living room. The child was absent because his mother just had a baby and needed help with household chores. The baby appeared to be well cared for and was approximately a week old. The dog also had five puppies that were squirming around the entire apartment. In the middle was a gas heater with a red tag from the Gas Company indicating it was condemned. There was a makeshift pipe leading to the outdoors through a broken window. This added to the chilly atmosphere in the apartment. The bathtub was full of clothes needing to be washed, and the water in the kitchen sink could only be turned on with a wrench.

I spoke to the mother about the school's concerns and told her I would follow up with getting her some assistance. Her primary concern was that her husband, a heavy drinker, would not appreciate any stranger coming to the house for any reason. I discussed a lot of her fears and promised to do what I could to make her life a little easier. Social services was able to step in and assist with finding appropriate safe housing.

Since well-baby visits were a priority with the city, I visited to demonstrate a safe baby bath and how to prepare and store formula. Formula preparation was a little different than open the can of powder, put in a scoop, add water, shake the bottle and give it to the baby. The milk had to be poured into prepared bottles that had to be sterilized along with the nipples. I demonstrated how to feed the baby properly, how to change the baby, and how to bathe the baby.

On one such call, I had to park my city car on the other side of a bustling multilane thoroughfare. I had a doll that I used for the demonstration of the bath. I had to carry my bag and doll across the street without dropping anything. With so many things to carry, I took the baby and shoved it under my arm. Across the street was a gas company work crew. One of the workers ran across the street, yelling, "Nurse, I'll take the baby for you." Then it dawned on me what that must have looked like. Here I am the model of how to take care of things as a public health nurse, and I've got a baby tucked under my arm like a football. I quickly explained this wasn't a real baby. Then I wondered how many other people saw that, and I thought, "I guess if it looks real, you have to treat it like it's real." I suppose I didn't make a really good impression that day.

That day I tried to explain to the mother how you needed to make sure the bottles were clean and washed in hot soapy water, rinsed, and allowed to dry. At that time, we boiled bottles to make sure they were sterile. I watched her older child crawl around the floor with formula in a bottle that still had orange juice residue in it. I doubted the mother would be adhering to sterile preparation after seeing the healthy child seemingly unaffected by a dirty bottle. I hoped she washed them better.

HUMANITY, OR LACK THEREOF, WILL NEVER CEASE TO AMAZE ME

I cared for a 17-year-old girl who had a baby and was thrown out of her house by her strict parents who would not accept the child out of wedlock. She was too young for public assistance, which started at eighteen, so she was on her own. She was able to find a lady who took her into her apartment in the rear of a barbershop in a somewhat sketchy neighborhood. There was no baby furniture and not a lot of baby supplies. The Salvation Army supplied her with some things for the baby but no crib. When I made my newborn baby visit, part of the City Charter in the City of Detroit, I was surprised at what I found. Since there was no baby crib, this new mama kept the baby in a dresser drawer, and when the baby cried, she closed the drawer. I could see I have a lot of education to do! I advised the new mom that babies need to breathe, and this was not a good idea. She felt this was safer for the baby than leaving the drawer open to being attacked by rats while she went through the neighborhood begging for food.

Her neighbors often supplied her with food, diapers, and formula for the baby. During the visit, this mom informed me she had chicken in the oven that was cooling down. I asked her how long it had been in there. She said a couple of hours. I told it was dangerous to leave the chicken out for several hours since it could develop into food poisoning. As I held the baby, she went to take the chicken out of the oven. When she opened the oven door, she screamed. I ran to the kitchen to see what was going on. There were two enormous rats eating the rest of the chicken.

I contacted some of the local churches, and I was able to find a woman who agreed to take the new mom and her baby into her home. She lived in Detroit in a nice neighborhood in a lovely brick house and provided this young mom with a home, a bedroom for the baby, and a crib, and things that she needed. I was gratified the teenager was able to manage a lot better. Later she was able to find part-time work filing. The lady she lived with was more than willing to be a babysitter. The mom and her child found the family she needed. This patient taught me that things are never as hopeless as they seem. At that moment, I learned a lot could be done with the right networking interventions.

THE NEIGHBORHOOD LOOKOUT

I often noted on my rounds that there would be somebody who would come up to my City car and say, "You go ahead, nurse, I'll watch your car for you." The community supplied the neighborhood watchman. As the neighborhood got to know me as the person who was helping them, they became my eyes and ears in the community. A lot of my families were two to three homes apart on the same block so, when I parked my car, by the time I reached the second home visit, they already knew I was coming.

I would take some time off and catch up on my nurses' notes at the Health Center. Handwritten notes were not allowed, so I needed to type my notes into the medical record. That's when I first met the gem of Northeast Health Center by the name of Giselle. She could type as fast as I could talk. It always amazed me that when I finished my dictation, she stopped typing and handed me the record complete with all the notes. She was an amazing individual and a skilled typist.

One day I had to call in an apartment building with the dwelling on the fourth floor. There were no elevators, just four flights of stairs. As I walked up those four flights, I encountered two gentle-men who were quite drunk. Both were armed and were arguing about who was going to shoot who. I thought, "Great, I need to pass them on the way going up and on the way going down, if they were still alive." They saw me, so there was no point in running out of the building.

As I passed them, they recognized me as a public health nurse. I smiled and said, "Be careful with guns because guns can really kill people." They laughed and said, "We know." The lady I was going to see met me at the head of the stairs and yelled at the fellows, "Get out of here!" I found this unnerving. I wasn't exposed to that a whole lot in the past and wasn't sure I wanted to be exposed to that a whole lot in the future!

When I got back to my car there was a bullet hole where someone dotted the "I" on the City of Detroit emblem. The neighborhood lookout wasn't available and thank goodness the car made a better target then I did. That's when my husband and I decided that I should go back to the hospi-tal; it was a lot safer. In all honesty I missed the hands-on patient care. The majority of my work with the Health Department was more medical social work than hands on nursing and I missed the nursing part. On to new adventures!

Chapter Seven

A Little Fish in a Big Pond, Journey Through the Cleveland Clinic

"And what nursing has to do in either case, is to put the patient in the best condition for nature to act upon him."

— Florence Nightingale

WHETHER YOU'VE HAD a little or a lot of experience, as a new graduate, you ask, "Should I work in a large healthcare system and be a little fish in a big pond, or am I better off being a big fish in a smaller pond?" The decision is based on several factors. A nurse with a bachelor's degree might be viewed as an expert on the latest philosophies in nursing practice. (That may not necessarily be true, but the perception is there; sometimes perception is far higher than the truth.)

On the other hand, if you chose to work in a large healthcare system's hospital, you can transfer to different nursing units without it affecting your seniority. If you don't like a nursing unit, you can transfer elsewhere within the hospital or even another hospital within that healthcare system. That can become a tremendous opportunity since you may not be sure where your passion lies within nursing unless you've been exposed to it.

Another consideration is where you would like to find yourself in five or ten years in the nursing profession? What is your ultimate goal?

- Is it a management position?

- Is it having advanced clinical skills?

- Is it certification, or even obtaining a higher degree?

Ask yourself, "What is my passion in this profession; what is it that makes me wake up in the morning and can't wait to get to work?" That's not realistic all the time. However, in any job, you will have good days and bad days. But what keeps you coming back is your interest in making those bad days better or turning them into good days. There is an old saying, "If you love what you do, you never really work a day in your life."

Moving to Cleveland, Ohio

The decision to move away from Detroit occurred when my husband, Ron, was accepted to the Ohio College of Podiatric Medicine in Cleveland, Ohio. The school has since merged with Kent State University and is part of their campus. I had the decision to make: where do I want to work in Cleveland? Should I select a small hospital in which my experience would make me a big fish in a little pond, or should I choose to work in a huge hospital system like the Cleveland Clinic and be a little fish in a big pond?

I started my nursing career in a small hospital that gave me the luxury of taking the time to get myself organized and improve my prioritization skills. Nursing practice was good old-fashioned standardized nursing practice. The patients received good care, but I did not give much thought into what I was doing for the patient. The physician staff had their routines that rarely changed. I was interested in research in some areas:

- What research took place?

- What were the results?

- Were the results valid?

- Or did somebody think they had a good idea and played with the numbers to make their project look better than what it was?

My small community hospital did not have research opportunities. My interest in research grew when I got to Cleveland. I didn't just want to *read about* what was the latest and greatest; I wanted to be *part of the process*. My interest centered around trauma, orthopedics, and the latest in heart disease. I applied to several smaller hospitals in the greater Cleveland area and decided to take a position at the Cleveland Clinic.

I was surprised to find out that the Cleveland Clinic preferred to hire new graduates, which was not the case in most hospitals, which wanted nurses with experience. The rationale for their decision was that new graduates do not come with bad habits learned elsewhere and could be easily trained to do it the way the Cleveland Clinic wants it done. (This makes sense when you think about it). The Cleveland Clinic was well known for its progressive research in several areas, including orthopedics.

The Cleveland Clinic subsidized my housing and offered free medical care to all employees and their families. That was a perk not mentioned at any facility. Because of the healthcare system's research, patients from all over the world came to experience advanced medical and surgical care.

Oh, My Aching Joints...We Can Fix That...Then and Now

I started my Cleveland Clinic journey on the orthopedic floor. (Chapter 4 describes orthopedics as "bedpan alley". I returned to the Cleveland Clinic version of bedpan alley.) Joint replacement was in its infancy during my employment at the Cleveland Clinic. Dr. John Charnley (1911-1982) pioneered the development of total hip arthroplasty in England. During the 1960s and partly the 1970s, orthopedic fellows went to England to observe and practice the techniques developed by Dr. Charnley. Occasionally he would come to the United States to lecture and demonstrate his research. Dr. Charnley was knighted in 1977 and became Sir John Charnley.

Patients suffering from hip misalignment, either from trauma, a congenital defect, or arthritis, flocked to the Cleveland Clinic for a total hip replacement. General criteria for patient selection was based on age, immobility, and significant pain.

Patients were at high risk for blood clots due to a lack of physical activity and mobility. The glue used at the time to cement in the prosthetic caused patients to have a high incidence of blood clot formation, therefore the majority of the patients were over 65 before they were considered a candidate for the surgery. The prosthetics were one-size-fits-all, yet the surgical outcomes were impressive.

Traction, Attraction, Distraction, and More Traction

In those early days, postoperative patients were on bed rest, traction, and a derotation strap glued to the leg preventing the external rotation of the leg after surgery. This caused a serious challenge to nursing care. It was difficult to reposition the patient due to the derotation strap as well as the patient's general immobility and pain. The sheets were changed from top to bottom rather than side to side. With the use of an over bed trapeze, patients were able to lift themselves a little to assist with any nursing care. Patients remained in traction for two to three weeks and, at times, required significant motivation to breathe deeply and do some minimal exercises such as foot and ankle pumps.

Our incentive spirometry bottles (an apparatus used to strengthen lungs and prevent the development of pneumonia) were not the same plastic creative devices we have today. I needed to construct an incentive spirometry bottle by using two empty glass IV bottles, some tubing, and a straw. The first bottle had water at the bottom, the tube was placed below the water level, and the patient was asked to blow through the straw, above the water level, causing enough pressure to move the water through the tubing to a second bottle. This was not easy!

Despite the work involved, it was so rewarding to see the patients who had been crippled, usually for many years, to get up and walk normally. One such memorable patient was a schoolteacher whose hip and leg were four inches shorter than the other leg. Many of the students would mercilessly tease her because of her severe limp. When she recovered from surgery, she went home able to wear two-inch heels and walk without a limp. She and the rest of us were in tears. What an incredible transformation from crippled to confident! There were so many stories like that.

In today's world, joint replacement surgery is considered elective and is a much better-organized program with a variety of choices of implantable components. Patients attend classes and know what to expect pre-op and post-op along with safety precautions such as using an elevated toilet seat, a walker, and aids for dressing. They learn to avoid stooping and bending to pick up things. Also, they realize it will take months to heal and become independently active as before surgery, only better.

Patients who undergo an anterior approach for hip joint replacement may not even need an elevated toilet seat. Rather than staying in traction for three weeks, patients go home in one day or even the day of surgery. Early discharge decreases the chance of hospital-borne organisms causing a major problem such as an infection destroying the new prosthetic. With home visits and outpatient physical therapy, patients do quite well.

'Your Heart Hurts? We Can Fix That Too' - Open Heart Surgery at the Cleveland Clinic

The Cleveland Clinic was at the forefront of open-heart surgery, repairing clogged coronary vessels and extending the life of many patients. I transferred to the surgical post-open-heart surgery unit, where we admitted patients either a day before their surgery or postop when they left the intensive care unit. Open-heart surgery was a relatively new venture and developed into a successful one. Since this was experimental, insurance did not cover it. Most of our patients paid cash. At the time, the open-heart procedures cost about $10,000, which is cheap, according to today's prices. But then again, what is your life worth?

One memorable patient was a new admission who decided to go down to the gift shop and purchase a newspaper. I was not finished with his admission process before he left the unit. Unfortunately, while in the elevator, he suffered a heart attack and became unresponsive. He had no identifiable wristband on so no one knew who he was, where he came from, or what his problem was. He was resuscitated and taken to the emergency room. Eventually, someone on the unit noticed that the patient was missing, and we all started to look for him.

From this experience, I learned the importance of putting a wristband on before the patient was undressed. In the event something happens off the unit, someone would know where this patient belongs. Today it's common practice to put the wristbands on the patients while in the admitting office before they even reach the unit. That memory stayed with me throughout my nursing career.

During my orientation to open-heart surgery, I had the pleasure of working with Dr. F. Mason Sones (1918-1985). Dr. Sones perfected the cardiac catheterization procedure. By injecting a small amount of dye and taking radiographic films, the dye outlined the coronary arteries and identified the location and degree of blockage, causing a lack of blood supply to the heart muscle.

Dr. Sones was an interesting individual who would spend a considerable amount of time explaining procedures to his patients. He had a great bedside manner. However, that didn't extend to his residents in training. He yelled a lot, but they learned a lot.

I later had an opportunity to meet a different Dr. Sones who cared for my sister's cardiac issues. I asked him if he, by any chance, had any relationship to Dr. F. Mason Sones at the Cleveland Clinic. He smiled and said, "As a matter of fact, that was my grandfather." Grandfather? Instantly I felt old. I have met a lot of *sons* of physicians I worked with over the years, but he was the first grandson old enough to be an attending physician in cardiology.

We had a lot of famous patients and dignitaries from foreign countries. One patient was a member of a royal family from one of the Middle Eastern countries. He was extremely handsome and brought his entourage of multiple wives and children and his own bodyguards. Our unit was also supplied with Secret Service individuals who protected the wing where his room was located. He did not interact a lot with the nurses but was more conversational with the physicians and residents.

One evening His Royal Highness had a temperature and was somewhat congested. It was my responsibility to notify the resident on-call for orders and possibly some diagnostic testing. After 5 PM, the surgical residents rotated, taking turns covering all the surgical patients in the hospital. You may or may not get the resident who's familiar with your patient's case. That was the issue here. The resident who responded to my request was a general surgery resident who was not familiar with the postoperative open-heart patients. When he came up to the unit, we told him the patient was a Crown Prince and needed to be treated like one. So, he told the security guards at the end of the hall and the Secret Service that he was the "Crown Prince of the Ozarks" and he wanted to see His Royal Highness. Therefore, they announced him in that manner.

The "Crown Prince of the Ozarks" came back to the desk, extremely embarrassed over acting like an idiot after he realized he saw an actual Crown Prince. It was a humbling moment for him and a good lesson to pay attention to what the nurses told him.

The resident ordered a chest x-ray, which required me to take His Royal Highness to the Radiology Department. I grabbed one of our wheelchairs and went down to his room and announced that I was taking him for a chest x-ray. One of the foot pedals fell, striking His Royal Highness on his ankle. He did not get hurt. One of his bodyguards flung himself to the floor, bowing continuously and saying something in their language. His reaction alarmed me. I asked my patient what was wrong with the bodyguard. His Royal Highness calmly looked at me, smiled, and said, "If this happened in my country, he probably would be, let's just say, *severely* disciplined." Great! I'm thinking, "How am I going to safely deliver my valuable patient to the Radiology Department, two floors down and three floors over, in this somewhat rickety wheelchair? No pressure there!" The Crown Prince's entourage joined us on the journey. We chatted briefly along the way; the patient safely returned to his room without any incident after the x-ray.

Upon His Royal Highness' return to his native country, he presented the open-heart surgeon with a beautiful Arabian stallion and a check for $10 million for open-heart surgery research at the Cleveland Clinic. This was a lovely gesture. However, there was no mention of the nursing staff who provided 24/7 nursing care. We didn't expect anything, but it would have been nice to be acknowledged in some small way.

Another interesting patient was the president of a large produce distribution business in Italy. He exported his fruit throughout Europe and the United States. He was upset when his sons sent him oranges that were not from his crop. I asked him, "How do you know they were not from your crop?" He turned the orange around to show me the Sunkist stamp. I guess his boys didn't think that he would turn the orange over.

The patient did well but needed a lot of encouragement to cough and deep breathe. During one of those encouraging moments, he coughed so hard the wires holding his sternum together popped, and his chest flung open. You could see his heart beating. We immediately put on a wet sterile dressing and rushed him back to the operating room. He spent the night in the intensive care unit and returned to us the following day. He shook his head, looked at us, and said, "I told you that wasn't a good idea." He healed well and returned to his home in Italy.

About a month after the Italian patient's discharge, a UPS driver showed up on my afternoon shift and asked me to sign for a package. We received 35 huge fruit baskets delivered from our gentlemen from Italy for all the nurses who took care of him. These were not little baskets. They contained whole pineapples, whole cantaloupes, and a bottle of wine in each one of the baskets. At that time, nurses were not supposed to accept gifts; however, what are you going to do with all the fruit? It would just spoil, not to mention, the wine might go bad. We sent our gratitude to Italy for his warm appreciation of the tender loving care we provided. What a lovely gesture!

A flamboyant Spanish patient came in for his open-heart surgery with a beautiful woman; we assumed she was his wife. She was extremely hands-on in comforting her poor, suffering husband. One day, a nurse's aides came running down the hall, yelling, "We got a problem." "What's the problem?" She informed me, "You know the lady who's in his room? That's not his wife. His wife is downstairs. She flew in from Spain to surprise him and boy, is she going to surprise him!" The real wife was on her way up to her husband's room; we had to grab his other "wife" and hide her before the real wife got on the unit. We just fixed the poor man's anatomy and didn't want anything to happen to him because of a domestic dispute. The mistress quickly left.

During my medication administration rounds one evening, a patient asked me if the pill I just gave him was an antibiotic. I didn't look it up, and I made the mistake of telling him I thought it was an antibiotic. Glaring at me, he said, "I am a pharmacist, and this is not an antibiotic." He suggested I look it up so I would know what to monitor my patient for and if the medication was effective. He added, "You should know the dose was appropriate before you give it." That was an extremely embarrassing moment. It was an anti-inflammatory drug and not an antibiotic. I assured him I knew what to monitor regarding the effects of the drug. I slithered out of the room. From that day forward, I never gave a medication with which I was unfamiliar. I knew the correct dosage, its intended result, and the side effects I needed to watch for.

My pharmacist patient made a good point. Physicians can make mistakes ordering medications or doses. So, when in doubt, look it up and clarify the dosage for the medication or the medication itself with the person who ordered it.

That makes a lot of sense. I recall an incident with an attending physician at the Cleveland Clinic. While making rounds, this attending handwrote an order for a medication. For the life of me, I couldn't decipher it despite all my experience and practice as a unit secretary. I called this attending physician at 10 PM and asked him what he wrote. He was agitated that I called him and asked why I didn't call one of his fellows or residents. I simply answered, "Why would I do that? They didn't write the order. You did." He contacted the nursing supervisor to inform me that there is a pecking order at the Cleveland Clinic, and I needed to be made aware of that. Okay, I promised not to bother him at night if he wrote better.

LIFE AFTER OPEN-HEART SURGERY - WE FIXED IT, NOW GO AHEAD AND LIVE

As I gained more experience in the postoperative unit, I realized the patient and family often did not understand the surgery and the difference it would make. They received a booklet the day before the patient went home. The booklet named the operation and included some of the postop information like follow-up appointments, new medications, and so on. The booklet also had information on emergency phone numbers and limitations, if any, on their activities postoperatively. In describing the actual heart surgery, the booklet used phrases and abbreviations such as "SVG (saphenous vein graft) to the LAD (left anterior descending artery) that was 80% obstructed". That meant absolutely nothing to the patient. Patients often also received incomprehensible explanations from the surgical resident what it meant.

At that time, CIBA Pharmaceuticals published a series of books, *Clinical Symposium*, illustrated by Frank Netter, MD. Frank Netter was a famous artist with a focus on various aspects of human anatomy. (In today's world, you can Google a picture of anything and get an illustration or an actual photograph.) His drawings were extremely accurate. One edition dealt with open-heart surgery and the use of coronary artery bypass grafts. I decided patients needed to have a good understanding of what type of surgery was done, what was repaired, and the fact that they were no longer cardiac cripples. Their problem was fixed.

I would gather the families and patients in one of the patient's rooms who was being discharged and do a presentation and explanation of their booklets. I explained that the saphenous vein graft (SVG) was a vein harvested from their leg that had similar properties to an artery. The vein was used to repair the 80% blocked left anterior descending artery (LAD) of the heart. When I showed them the pictures of the main vessels of the heart, they had a much better understanding of what was repaired. They understood their circulation was excellent, and when they went home, they could live a normal life without fear of crushing chest pain or having another heart attack, as long as they followed their doctor's orders. My presentations became quite popular with the patients and their families.

One evening, one of the heart surgeons stood in the doorway and listened to one of my presentations. I did not know he was there. He was impressed and said, "This is great that the patients know what we did and that they're going to be okay now."

I was pleased to find out that to this day, the Cleveland Clinic still has a similar postoperative class for patients to understand the impact of their heart surgery and what to expect in the future. It makes me feel great! I think the patients will be more compliant if they understand the why and what regarding their surgery. The *Clinical Symposium* pictures were a great help. Most patients didn't even know that the heart is located under the sternum. My nursing skills were more effective than the teaching of the residents, who often had limited English.

A position opened in the operating room, and I figured that this was an opportunity for me to see if I like the OR. On to another venture in nursing!

Chapter Eight

Challenges of the Operating Room and How to Deal with Quirky People

"OMG! A surgeon almost died in front of me today!!! But then I counted to 10, put the scalpel back on the mayo stand. He never even knew."

—Anonymous

My interest in orthopedics led me to the operating room where a position opened for the manager in the orthopedic section at the Cleveland Clinic Department of Surgery. I like the thought of going back to working the day shift; I decided to give it a whirl.

Operating room (OR) nursing is very different from any other nursing form. It has its own set of skills and much-needed personality to manage the participants – surgeons, the staff, the patients before anesthesia, and their little quirks.

Many of the surgeons had a God complex because their general thought was "to cut is to cure." The results were immediate rather than waiting for a medication to go into effect to see any results. One could almost understand that philosophy since immediate surgical intervention saved a lot of lives. However, the nursing care and compliance by the patient kept them from a repeat performance in the OR.

Working in the OR took me back to my candy striper days, and thinking surgeons wore gloves so as not to leave fingerprints. Now I realize they wore masks maybe for the same reason – anonymity.

SAME CIRCUS, DIFFERENT CLOWNS

All surgeons have a similar personality. One OR nurse described the operating room as "the same circus but different clowns." I worked with orthopedic surgeons who were mostly carpenters. Urologists were the plumbers, and the neurosurgeons were Gods, at least in their minds.

Each surgeon had a card that identified the size of the gloves, their preference for sutures, extras for certain cases, and so on. The scrub nurse is responsible for all equipment to be working and present. The sharps (blades) should be sharp. The scrub nurse had to replace missing articles or anything that wasn't perfect or let Central Supply Room (CSR) know so they can make the case carts complete. It was the circulating nurse's job to document who was in the room, assist with sharps, sponge, and instrument counts, and to fetch any additional or missing supplies during the procedure.

Even when things are ready to go for any procedure, the unexpected can happen. One such incident involved a patient having minor elbow procedure. When the surgeon moved the overhead lamp for a better light angle, the glass fell out, striking the patient and cutting his knee. After surgery, the patient woke up and couldn't figure out why his knee hurt. He expected to have elbow pain. When we told him what happened, he was grateful the glass didn't result in a second circumcision.

Patients were generally pre-medicated on the nursing unit before being sent down to the OR. As a staff nurse, I remember giving a lot of those medications in the preop holding area because

I didn't notice my patient had left for the OR. Eventually, my timing got a lot better.

The preop holding area had an interesting array of stretchers separated by a curtain. (In today's world, the patients do not arrive the night before surgery but usually within a couple of hours before the scheduled procedure. This allows for the patient to be seen by the anesthesiologist, have the IV started, and go through a regular checklist to make sure everything is ready. That wasn't necessarily the case in my early OR experiences.) The preop holding area was also known as the "snoring" zone. Once the patients were pre-medicated they slept. What else would they do?

Some of the patients needing minor procedures arrived on the day of surgery and were seen for clearance in the preop holding area by the anesthesiologist.

An incident occurred when two ladies, neighbors, appeared in the preop holding area at the same time. Judy recognized Betty and wanted to know what procedure she was having. Betty was having a polyp removed from her nose, nothing terribly exciting or embarrassing. The only privacy available was a curtain drawn between the stretchers, which did not allow for a confidential review of past medical/surgical history by the anesthesiologist. Reviewing Betty's surgical history, the anesthesiologist commented that Betty had an abortion when she was young. The next thing we heard was Judy yelling at Betty, "How could you do that; how could you kill a child?" That exchange was awkward for both parties. After surgery, they may have remained neighbors, but I'm not sure they remained friends. Some of these awkward moments could have been avoided if the anesthesiologist was more concerned about maintaining patient privacy and spoke in a much lower tone.

'It's A Good Thing the Patient Is Asleep and Didn't Hear That' ... and Other Stories of the OR

Some surgeons liked music to help them focus while they operated. The range went from acid rock, opera, classical, jazz, and the blues. Some worked in quiet; some told stories and jokes, and some discussed their love lives. Some of the jokes and stories could be considered off-color but were funny. They reduced the stress in the room and often were entertaining.

At times, the OR staff acted as counselors for the surgeons. I often wondered if the surgeons were paying attention to the procedure. I observed lots of drama at times. It takes quite a sense of humor, dedication, and patience to work in the OR. I have plenty of that.

Nurses often took the brunt of the surgeon's frustration. That was the case with Dr. Tipton, one of our orthopedic surgeons. When Dr. Tipton started to yell at the nurses, one of the OR nurses I worked with would tickle his ankle to bring him back to reality. I wasn't sure if that works with everybody, but it did work with Dr. Tipton. It is hard to yell at anyone when you're laughing.

One compelling case involved a Minor Procedure Room incident of a patient having some lumps and bumps removed. The patient had belongings under the cart. His cell phone was set to record the sounds in the OR. The phone recorded the surgeon's comments about the patient during the procedure. They weren't very flattering! The surgeon used some choice names describing the patient's personality or lack thereof. Referring to the patient as a hypochondriac, the surgeon further inferred that all the patient needed was a better sex partner than his current wife. The patient was horrified after he heard the tape. Later the patient sued the doctor for slanderous comments. I don't know the outcome of the lawsuit, but it pays to keep your words sweet because you never know when you may have to eat them.

How to Dodge Instruments and Other Terrifying Moments In the OR

As the nurse manager for the Orthopedic Surgery Section, my job was to occasionally observe some of the cases to make sure my department was running smoothly. I received complaints about one temperamental orthopedic surgeon, Dr. Cooley, who had a bad habit of throwing dull saw blades over his shoulder. I decided to observe one of his cases one day and that was exactly what happened. I was standing in the back of the room, and there was a lot of discussion with the residents about the procedure in progress. Suddenly, following numerous expletives, a surgical saw blade came whizzing my way. It just missed me. I started to rethink my career in the OR. I fancy myself as a rather easy-going person who has no tolerance for bad behavior or incompetence. I don't mean to infer that Dr. Cooley was incompetent, but he sure had bad behavior.

I could not tolerate bad behavior and decided to leave the operating room and return to my awake patients and families. I missed the opportunity to do patient/family teaching and meeting the needs of those patients and families in a safer environment. Dr. Cooley came to the nursing unit and apologized for his behavior and asked me to return to the OR. I was tempted; I liked the teamwork, but I opted for my awake patients. At least I had the experience, and what an experience it was.

Our afternoon supervisor, Ms. Jean Reynolds, had a friend who was director of nursing at one of our smaller community hospitals run by an HMO. She was looking for a competent nurse who could serve as relief supervisors on the off shifts. Miss Reynolds approached me since she recognized my talent and interpersonal relationships skills. Why not explore another avenue of nursing? I took her up on the challenge. I always wanted to know what it would be like to be the boss... I was about to find out!

Chapter Nine:

Supervision Can Be Scary

*"Rejoice in your work; never lose sight
of the nursing leader you are now and
the nursing leader you will become."*

— Sue Fitzsimmons, PhD, RN

After leaving the operating room, I returned to my post open heart surgery unit and was glad to see my patients again. One afternoon while I was on duty, Ms. Reynolds, our afternoon nursing supervisor, approached me to help her with some part-time supervision at one of our HMO community hospitals. I was flattered she recognized my managerial abilities, so I took her up on her offer. My husband was still in school, and the extra money would come in handy. I wondered, "How bad could this be to work as a supervisor? After all, I'm a good nurse, I'm an experienced nurse, and I can certainly guide others to do their best." This hospital was small, approximately 50 beds, and was a part of a large HMO based in California. The hospital had an emergency room and medical and surgical units. It was one of the first managed-care organizations in the country and is now the largest managed care organization in the United States.

The staff was permanent with not too many new hires or inexperienced nurses. One of the nurses, I will call her Clara, was 86 years old and still working as a nurse. Clara had taught English in Africa and nursing. An experienced nurse, Clara knew what to do and how to do it and came across as coldly efficient. But she did work hard and insisted everybody else did who worked with her.

My role was relief supervisor on the midnight shift. Interacting with professionals on a different level took a little adjusting. Most of the individuals I supervised were at least twice my age, and I could read their faces: "What could *she* possibly know? However, she came from the Cleveland Clinic; therefore, she must be smart. Let's see just how smart she is."

I prepared myself for the new role by thinking of what I would do in case of an emergency such as a fire, a cardiac arrest, or a disturbance in the emergency room. I thought I was ready. Throughout my whole nursing career, I was acutely aware of the "what if's" and somewhat prepared for all those unexpected emergencies that can throw your day off and your *career* off as well.

On my first shift, I made frequent rounds, introduced myself to the staff, and gave my pager number if they needed anything. I stopped by the emergency room and introduced myself to the physician, and things seem to be stable for the moment.

WHERE'S THE FIRE?

That didn't last long. One of the nurses' aides made toast for a patient. Unfortunately, the toaster was directly underneath the heat sensor, and the fire alarms went off. Everyone knows that when a fire alarm goes off, you don't take the elevator. So I didn't; I ran down the stairs and out of the door to find myself, not on the first floor, but outside in pitch-black darkness. I did not know where the front door was since this was my first time at the hospital. Thankfully the door is alarmed, so somebody heard the alarm and decided to look for me as I stumbled my way in the darkness. I will never again do that without a flashlight.

I soon found myself at the front door and met the Cleveland Fire Department staff, who asked me, "Where was the fire?" I told them I didn't call, and there was no fire. They informed me the hospital was directly wired to the fire department, and when the sensor goes off, it shows up as a fire. They automatically respond. Good idea, I wish somebody had told me that; I learned another lesson.

After a quick inspection, the firefighters came back to the hospital within 5 minutes and told me, "You called us again.". I didn't call them the first time. I wanted to whine, "Don't be mad at me." I didn't know the alarm system had to be reset, and of course, that was one of those things I did not find out in advance. The reset was locked up in the switchboard, to which I had no access. A grumpy fireman gained access, showed me how to reset the fire alarm, and advised me to move the toaster. I did, and things quieted down for the night.

After supervising a few more times, I quickly gained the respect of the staff. I helped when they needed an extra pair of hands. I provided additional staff where and when it was necessary. My first concern was patient safety and delivering the best care that we could considering any limitations.

One day my emergency room aide, who was generally efficient and cheerful, came into work in a fog. I asked her what was wrong, and she said,

"Nothing" and moved on with her duties. I sensed she wasn't candid, and something was bothering her. I couldn't put my finger on it, and she was not willing to talk to me.

About 5 AM, the Cleveland Police came in and asked if she was on duty. I told them she was, and they came to arrest her for murder. I was shocked! They told me she had killed her husband before coming to work. I couldn't believe it. "You've got to kidding." They told me her husband was abusive, and she had a restraining order. He showed up drunk, threatening her with a baseball bat. She used a shotgun to blow him off the front porch, left the body in the bushes, and came to work. I guess that would make you a little distant at work. She was arrested later to be released as the police officers viewed her actions as self-defense. She fully believed, as did the police, had her husband gained access to the house, he would have killed her.

I liked supervision, and the staff responded well to my guidance. In 1973, a full-time supervision opportunity came up for me to work at Mothers' General Hospital in Cleveland. Mothers' General Hospital was originally founded as a women's and children's free medical and surgical dispensary. It was the only hospital in Cleveland founded by two women physicians, the first women to practice medicine in Cleveland.

This was a seven-story hospital with an active medical staff of 52 and departments of surgery, medicine, gynecology, pediatrics, radiology, anesthesiology, and pathology. When the obstetric unit closed, a women's alcoholic rehabilitation unit opened with the help of a federal grant and as the only alcoholic rehabilitation unit just for women in the state.

The hospital also had an emergency room and an intensive care unit. I remember seeing the last OB patient as she was being discharged. She was a Hungarian woman who delivered twins. The discharge process looked rather pitiful; mom held the babies one in each arm, dad had all the bags and two bunches of roses, and everybody was crying, mom, the babies, and dad. I hope they all survived.

I worked the midnight shift and occasionally the afternoon shift, if needed. Supervision provided me with an opportunity to educate staff to work smarter rather than harder. One of the things I stressed with my staff was to know the emergency procedures. I remembered my experiences with the fire alarms at the HMO hospital. When you're in a path of a tornado, you don't have the time to look up what you should be doing. What if the power goes off and you have a ventilator patient?

How long do you think you could keep squeezing that Ambu bag before your arms give out?

I often annoyed the staff with my question: "What would you do if you found this basket on fire right now?" It was interesting to hear some different responses. At least I got them questioning, "What would I do?" In my heart, I felt I was at least preparing them to save themselves and the patients in the event of an emergency.

'Humor Me, Do It My Way'

The hospital had several unions: RNs, LPNs, Maintenance, Dietary Department, and security. As the only supervisor on duty on the off shift, I was responsible for everyone's activities. I couldn't possibly remember all the different union contracts and the issues involved with stewards and unions in general during my first experience working with a variety of unions. But I remembered something about the "rights of management" clause which is incorporated in every contract.

I believe that majority of the union members I dealt with had lost their contracts or were not very aware of the content. When something needed to be done, I would simply remind them of the "rights of management" clause in their union contract gave me the authority to reassign anyone to temporary duties based on patient needs. After all, we were hospital staff and needed to provide safe patient care. No one ever challenged me on that "rights of management" argument. That one statement allowed me to keep order and the facility smoothly functioning.

As the supervisor, I had keys to all the departments. Around 6 AM, the dietary department would come to get the keys to the kitchen. One morning, the dietary staff came and asked for the keys for the morgue. Now, this piqued my curiosity, so I took the keys and went with her wondering why she needed the keys to the morgue. She explained to me they ran out of room in the refrigerator, so the afternoon cook put two pans of Jell-O in the morgue. It was refrigerated. I could not believe they did that. (I can't eat Jell-O in a hospital to this day wondering where it was stored.) I told the dietary manager about the novel storage idea; she was horrified. I guess I wasn't the only one who learned something that day.

What Were You Thinking?

Mothers' General Hospital was an old building with its heating system operated by a boiler that required constant pressure maintained at a certain level for safety. That duty was the responsibility of a maintenance worker named Frank Jones. Frank was a Vietnam veteran with a drinking problem. Looking back on his personality, I realize he probably suffered from post-traumatic stress disorder. His responsibility was to maintain the boiler pressure so the building wouldn't blow up. This is one of those jobs you take very seriously. I would occasionally visit the Maintenance Department to make sure things were okay and to see if anybody needed anything. I was, after all, responsible for the entire building.

On several occasions, when I visited Frank, he was sound asleep. I woke him up, gave him a warning that his lack of attention to his job put us all in danger. He was disgruntled when I woke him up. "I realize this job may be boring, but the safety issue affected everybody," I told him. During one of those visits, I found Frank asleep again and the boiler making all sorts of noises. Again, I woke Frank up, but this time I also called his boss, who came in and immediately fired him. He said the level of pressure was so high in the boiler that it may have exploded. That got my attention.

Several days later, I was working the midnight shift and received a call about 1 AM from the switchboard operator informing me that someone had called her and said that there was a bomb in the hospital. Now there's a problem I never expected. I immediately called the Cleveland Police Department and told them that I had just received a bomb threat. The officer I spoke with suggested I look around to see if I find anything that looks suspicious. If I found something, don't touch it and call him back. In my innocence, I thought maybe *they* would come and help me look.

I grabbed the security guard, Danny, and the two large rings with about 120 keys and started our hunt. The facility did not have one master key; every locked door had its own key. I began to wonder, "Who would want to blow us up?" I considered our former boiler operator, Frank, who was recently fired and didn't like me.

It was an impossible task to check every single locked room in a 7-story building. The bomb could be anywhere. I remembered that the maintenance department also had the same set of keys.

I decided to start our search in the Maintenance Department. That would make the most sense rather than hiding a bomb in someone's locked office. After all, Frank didn't like his boss either. Danny and I went down to Maintenance and started looking around. We both separated and met at the manager's office. It was hard to tell if anything was out of place. Then I noticed a white box with a red painted cross on the lid. It was next to the chairs where the manager met with people.

I called the police department back and informed them we indeed found a suspicious package that might be a bomb. "What's our next step?" The bomb squad and the fire department showed up within minutes. They opened the box and found a couple of sticks of dynamite and a clock that Frank had wired to the explosives. "Would this go off "? I asked. "Absolutely, yes!" I couldn't believe that anybody would do something like that to a hospital. However, Frank was not in his right mind. Frank's background in the military was in demolition, so he knew how to carry out his plans. No matter how much I preach to my staff about being ready for emergencies, this is one that astonished me. How could you ever be prepared for something like this?

Remember the patient at the Cleveland Clinic who had a heart attack on the elevator, and nobody knew who he was because he had no identification wristband? (See Chapter 7). A similar situation occurred at Mothers' General Hospital, involving the nursery. One of our fire alarms sounded, and the nurse working the nursery thought she smelled smoke. She opened a blanket, took all the babies out of the bassinets, put them on the blanket, and dragged the blanket across to the other side of the fire doors. She was able to handle all of the babies. However, some of them did not have identifying bracelets, which were often taped to the head of the bassinets when they came off. We had baby footprints, and with the help of a forensic pathologist, hopefully, we matched them to the right baby. There was no fire, just the alarm that sounded. I often wondered if the right baby went home to the right family. Another important lesson learned: make sure everybody is identifiable.

WHERE'S THE CAP?

We had a group of physicians who insisted on using ether to remove adhesive or any other sticky surface on the patient. Ether can explode if not properly stored or used. One time Dr. Isle, a 92-year-old surgeon, used ether to remove a 6-inch-wide tape triple wrapped around the patient's pelvis to stabilize a fracture. Unfortunately, the staff lost the cap, and everybody was getting a little sleepy or nauseated from the ether. They called me since I was the supervisor, but I didn't know what to do either. I thought the best thing to do would be to call the fire department. That made sense since they are accustomed to working with flammables/explosives and could advise me as to what to do with the ether.

The firemen I spoke with suggested I take it up on the roof and pour it into a metal bedpan and just let it evaporate. He also asked me why we didn't have a trap can to store the ether. I didn't know what that was, but I'm sure there probably was one in the OR, someplace. The following morning, I received a phone call from the administrator because the Battalion Chief Cleveland Fire Department showed up on his doorstep and wanted to know why we didn't have a spring-loaded pressure can to store ether because that was required by law. The administrator wanted to know why I didn't call him. In the middle of the night, I didn't think he would know what to do. I thought I did what made sense.

Other incidents might make you scratch your head. It was a policy of the hospital that if any packages arrived after 5 PM when their office was closed, a message was left for the supervisor to accept the package and place it where it needed to go. One Friday afternoon shift about 5 PM, UPS delivered a rather heavy large box marked "perishable". I told the driver that I was not to accept any packages without notification from the manager of the department. The driver informed me that these were radioisotopes requested on an emergency basis, and he wasn't going to take it back. I called the Radiology Department head, and there was no answer. The UPS driver was kind enough to place the large, heavy box into a wheelchair for me.

I headed for the radiology department but did not find any special area marked for radioisotopes.

They did have a refrigerator, and since the box was marked perishable, I took out a shelf and slid the box into the refrigerator. It barely fit, but I was able to close the door. The following morning, I went shopping since that was my usual routine for Saturday mornings. When I arrived home, my husband said, "Call the hospital immediately. They are in a panic looking for you. What did you do with the radioisotopes? They can't find them." The Radiology staff was concerned because children were playing around the hospital might have found the radioisotopes.

I called the hospital and informed them that I place my perishables in the refrigerator, and they should look in their refrigerator. I found out the "perishable" part was due to the half-life, not spoilage. If they had informed me of the shipment, and where to store it, we wouldn't be having this conversation. Everybody was safe. Another lesson learned: keep the communication going!

ARE YOU CHECKING YOUR EYELIDS FOR CRACKS OR SLEEPING?

My employees knew they could depend on me when situations got out of hand or when they just needed some extra help. We shared a mutual respect. Anyone with experience working night shift knows that it's sometimes difficult to stay awake. The hours are almost inhumane. However, patients are sick during the night and need someone to take care of them.

One nurse amazed me. She would stand behind the door with her knees locked, propped up in the corner, close her eyes, and could sleep standing up like a horse. I nudged her a little, and she almost fell like a tree; she was headed that way. She came to and said she was just resting her eyes for a minute.

While making rounds in the intensive care unit, I discovered one nurse was on her break and away from the unit, and the charge nurse, Helen Gaines, was sitting at the desk with her eyes closed. I stood there for a few minutes; she wasn't moving. I asked her if she was sleeping or if she was checking her eyelids for cracks. She said she was just resting her eyes because she was exhausted that day. I warned her, "This is an intensive care unit, which means you must continuously monitor patients." I checked her patients; they were stable. I gave her a verbal warning and told her, "There will be greater consequences if I find you asleep again. An intensive care unit is an area where you need to stay awake". She again claimed that she was not sleeping.

Unfortunately, my issues with Ms. Gaines continued. She was the only nurse in the ICU on a specific night. ICU had only two patients that night – both patients were monitored and were stable. While making my rounds, I noticed Ms. Gaines was again asleep at the desk; however, at this time, both patients' cardiac monitor alarms were ringing. They did not wake her up. That concerned me. I evaluated the patients, adjusted their alarms, and then spoke to Ms. Gaines. I sent her home. That left me with no ICU nurse.

I contacted the Director of Nursing that night; she suggested transferring the patients to Olympia Hospital, where the cardiologist was also on staff. They had more beds and more nursing staff available. I transferred both patients to Olympia Hospital, and when the cardiologist made rounds in the morning, he was livid: "Why were my patients moved?" I explained to him they were moved because there was no staff to take care of them. He did not believe me. He made a formal complaint to Administration. The administrator supported my decision and terminated Ms. Gaines.

Ms. Gaines later filed a discrimination suit in Federal Court through the labor union. However, she did not win. She lost her appeal, and the judge agreed she was guilty of dereliction of duty by her lack of patient observation and sleeping while on duty.

Your Lack of Planning Is Not My Emergency!

The managers were responsible for staffing the units based on acuity, the census, and the needs of their patients. That sounds like a reasonable request, and it was. Occasionally someone would call in sick, and then it became the managers' responsibility to cover the short staffing issue. What usually happened was they were unable to locate anyone to come in and cover. The administration expected the manager to come in and cover the shift and have the next day off.

The other option I had in handling short-staffing was to transfer the patients again or work the unit myself. While I didn't mind helping with patient care, it was difficult to manage the enterprise and take full responsibility for a group of patients.

I had one unpleasant encounter with Dr. Adams, who was our cardiologist. Dr. Adams insisted that there be two nurses in the ICU/CCU at all times, even if we had one patient. In a way, I could understand that rationale. If one nurse gets tied up with a critical patient, the other nurse can get help or assist. I could not leave two nurses in the unit with one stable patient to be transferred the next day. So, I pulled one nurse to the surgical unit, which was absolutely swamped and short-staffed. She immediately called the cardiologist to complain. Dr. Adams came to my office to complain. I very politely informed him, "When you sign the checks for those nurses, you can place them wherever you'd like. As long as the hospital signs their checks and mine, we all have a job to do, and it will be done expeditiously and with keeping patient safety in mind." You can imagine how well that went over. After a few minutes, he backed off and said, "Too bad; you do what you have to do."

Supervision can be tough at times. I filled in the gaps when I could both in the intensive care unit and particularly in the emergency room. I always supervised and taught in some fashion, no matter where I worked. That was part of just me being a nurse. When you delegate the task, you must supervise. You have the responsibility when you ask someone to do something to make sure that is done correctly and promptly. This is the basis of nursing practice. As a nurse, there's a lot of things I was interested in and situations I wanted to try to see if I liked it.

The year before my husband graduated, we had our first child, my daughter Hollie. She was a very good baby. I was working full-time on the midnight shift as the nursing supervisor. Balancing sleeping time and the work schedule was challenging at best. My neighbor occasionally helped keep an eye on Hollie while I caught up with some badly needed sleep. My husband came home from school around 4 PM, which allowed me to get at least five hours of sleep before I went to work. Life soon became a juggling act between school, my work schedule, and occasionally his clinical rotations. We managed! It was a challenging year.

Hollie slept through the night from the first day I brought her home from the hospital. I remember calling the pediatrician and asking him if I should wake her up to feed her. His response was simple, "Are you kidding me? If she's asleep, let her sleep. She will let you know when she's hungry." I was no different than any new mother; babies didn't come with directions. My mother was in another state, but only a phone call away for advice. We drove back to Michigan several times to visit with the family and pick up some food from my dad (remember he was a butcher).

My husband finally graduated in 1975 from medical school as a podiatrist. I had a special graduation present for my husband. I found out that morning that I was pregnant with our second child, our son Ryan. My husband had just graduated, was ready to start his residency, and move back home to Michigan. Our family was growing.

My grandmother suggested we live with her since she was alone and wanted company and couldn't wait to help with her great-grandchildren. This opportunity allowed us to save money for a home when Ron completed his residency. We took her up on her generous offer, packed up our little family, and moved back to Michigan. I was looking forward to seeing my family and my friends as well as finding a job opportunity back home. I considered possibly returning to the afternoon shift as a nursing supervisor to allow me time in the morning to get Hollie settled and spend some time with the family before going to work. Ron was busy during the day and took over keeping daughter entertained and ready for bed in the evening. My grandmother was a great help and enjoyed watching the little one grow.

CHAPTER TEN:

BACK TO SUPERVISION AND THE EMERGENCY ROOM

"Leadership is not about being in charge. Leadership is about taking care of those in your charge."

—Simon Sinek

MY HUSBAND GRADUATED in 1975 and I moved back to Michigan. I was hired at Northwest General Hospital, a community hospital. They had approximately 300 beds and most of the employees working were within walking distance of the hospital. I lived about a mile away and on a nice day I would walk to work. I was hired as the afternoon nursing supervisor and was looking forward to starting yet another adventure in management.

I soon remembered as the supervisor the buck stopped with me. If there were staffing issues, I solved them. My biggest responsibility was to maintain a safe patient environment, to educate my staff, and generally help where an extra pair hands was needed. I enjoyed working the afternoon shift since it allowed me to sleep in, Hollie permitting, in the morning, run errands, and still arrive on time to work.

Like any hospital, we had our share of personalities who at times were difficult. Those personalities weren't limited to the patients and their families. An incident occurred when Dr. Mark Peters locked horns with one of my nurses. Dr. Peters was an excellent physician who at times liked to grandstand and berate the nursing staff in the presence of visitors. He had a very loud voice. Most the nurses would avoid him like the plague when they saw him coming on the unit.

On one such occasion I had asked Dr. Peters to join me in my office. Unwillingly he did and we had a little conversation. I told him I was going to tell him something his mother did not tell him. He looked rather puzzled. I simply told him that if he had a complaint he needed to bring it to me, the supervisor, rather than yelling at the nurses at the desk. This made them look incompetent and was not comforting to visitors or patients who could hear his booming voice. His mother should have told him he was born with a placenta just like the nurses and not a pedestal. He really wasn't in agreement and stormed out of my office. I hoped he got the message.

REMEMBER ME?

As luck would have it, Dr. Peters became ill and needed to be hospitalized. Normally any hospital would have a private "VIP" room for such a patient. However, the census was rather full, and the private rooms were used for isolation. Dr. Peters' doctor admitted him to a semiprivate room on the floor where he previously antagonized the nursing staff. Besides being sick, I think he was actually scared.

To my amazement, Dr. Peters called me and asked me to come to his bedside since the nurse he yelled at frequently needed to start an IV and he thought I would do a better job. I'm not so sure I would have done a better job since the nurses on the unit started a lot more IVs than I did as a supervisor. I spoke to the nurse and she assured me that she would be professional and wouldn't hurt him on purpose. However, she was hoping his attending physician would order maybe an enema or two or something that would be far more gratifying than just starting an IV.

When I visited Dr. Peters, I assured him that my nurses were quite competent and would have no problem starting his IV. During my visit, his nurse came in and started the IV with no difficulty at all. He was grateful for my presence, just in case. It was amazing how his personality changed once he returned to work and how nice he was to the staff. He even brought them cookies to thank them for their tender loving care. It may help every healthcare provider to be a patient at least once. The view is very different from the other side.

To Shave or Not to Shave, That Is the Question...

Being a patient for a physician can be very challenging. This was the case for Dr. Cranston, who was Chief of Medical Services and director of our employee health clinic. The whole staff knew Dr. Cranston, a kindhearted elderly gentleman. Dr. Cranston's doctor admitted him the night before his scheduled urology surgery and ordered a surgical prep. This entailed shaving Dr. Cranston's body from his nipples to his knees. The purpose of the prep is to make sure no loose hairs get into a surgical site and could possibly cause an infection. There was a problem, however. Because Dr. Cranston was so familiar with the entire staff all my nurses refused to do this extensive shave, which included his groin.

Remember that comment about the buck stops with me? It did again, and I was elected to play barber. The unit was busy, and I didn't mind helping but this was an awkward moment for me as well as for my staff. I shaved a lot of patients in the ER. My reputation was on the line.

I gathered all the necessary equipment, a couple of towels shaving kits, and proceeded to Dr. Cranston's room. I visited him earlier but did not expect to be his barber. I put on my best professional demeanor and informed him that I was going to get him ready for surgery. He seemed less than thrilled and we chatted about various things like the weather, how his grandchildren were doing, and other stuff that came to my mind to lessen the awkwardness. The prep was going quite well until I got down to some rather delicate private areas, which I managed to nick. I apologize profusely and Dr. Cranston just smiled and suggested that the prep could possibly be finished in the OR since he might want to use some of those parts again. I fully understood and agreed. At least I tried, boy did I try!

It's Always Busy in the ER

As the nursing supervisor I spent a lot of time helping in the emergency room. The afternoon shift was always the busiest. Working in the emergency room (ER) has always been of special interest to me. Your patients come, and they go; they do not stay any longer than 24 hours at the most. You also avoid the politics of teamwork on the nursing units, nor do get involved with some patients that seem to stay forever along with their annoying families.

In the ER patients come in to be treated for whatever is bothering them. It's also exciting to see who is coming through your doors next, you learn to assess and prioritize very rapidly. One of our emergency physicians, Dr. Anayo, took great pride in guessing what was wrong with the patient just by looking at them. He had a talent for diagnosis and was usually correct.

As a nurse, I was always eager to assist the physician in the practice of his duties as well as anticipate those needs. It was a real camaraderie in the ER, just like the OR. With the right staff on duty, it was an example of real-time teamwork in action. I knew ahead of time what everybody thought before they had to say it. I kept the patients moving through the department as fast as I could.

At times it became difficult for the receptionist writing up the patient to truly understand when they had to be seen immediately for a real emergency or it can wait until a bed was available.

An incident involved the patient who came with a terrible headache, sore throat and general symptoms of the flu. Not exactly an emergency but I'm sure the patient felt miserable. The secretary ran back and told us that we had to see her immediately because she was in bad shape. Our beds were filled, and we really had no place to put the patient; consequently, I saw her while she was in a wheelchair. She had the flu, and I explained to the receptionist that this is not a life-and-death matter, it just feels like it.

Shortly after that a young gentleman came in with a stab wound to the chest. It was a small hole, but the patient did have blood dripping down his chest. The receptionist thought it would be nice to sop up the blood and have him just put a little pressure on the site. So, she came into the ER and grabbed a handful of paper towels. I thought maybe somebody vomited and needed cleaning up or whatever until a bed was ready. I followed her. I took one look at this rather cyanotic young man whose head was back up against the wall trying to hold onto paper towels on his stab wound. I quickly informed the receptionist; this is an emergency! I got him back as soon as possible and quickly took him into the trauma room after moving one of the patients into a wheelchair. The doctor and a thoracic surgeon immediately saw him, ordered stat chest x-rays, and took him to the

OR for the repair of a collapsed lung and internal bleeding. Although the hole in his chest was small, the damage wasn't.

THE FREQUENT FLYERS

Our local fire department had a real sense of humor. One of their favorite tricks was to bring a semi-conscious patient on 100% oxygen by mask, place them on a stretcher, and then take off. Once we took the mask off, I realized the patient was semi-conscious due to being extremely intoxicated, better-known as dead drunk. The oxygen didn't wake him up, it just covered the odor of the alcohol. I had the pleasure of dealing with the aftermath of too much booze, and instant replay of his last meal. Usually, I was prepared for that but not always, so I learned to carry a second pair of shoes when I went to work.

Like any emergency room, we had our share of frequent flyers every Friday. When the bars closed, our business picked up. I could almost predict who was coming in and what to expect. The routine usually consisted of finding a quiet dark spot where they could sober up before they went home or to jail, whichever came first. Our Police Department was very friendly and would often take some of our frequent flyers home. One such patient, Phil, would rather go to jail than incur the wrath of his wife after he "drank" his paycheck and came home with the police. Suddenly jail did not look so bad.

One Friday evening, the Detroit Police brought in a gentleman from a local bar fight. This was not an unusual occurrence since the city had a bar on just about every block. This bar was on the border of Detroit and a neighboring city. Therefore, the officers angrily debated which Police Department was responsible for the paperwork. The gentleman had a small laceration above his eye near the temple area. It wasn't bleeding much, and he was breathing. His vital signs were stable, but he was not verbally responsive. He vomited, not unusual, so we placed them in an observation area to have him sleep it off since we had more pressing emergencies to deal with at the time.

When I went to check on him, he was dead. I contacted the medical examiner to pick up the body and called both Police Departments to figure out the name of the dead patient and who would take control of the case.

The next day I received a phone call from the homicide division, Detroit Police Department wanted to know the name of the physician and staff who tended to our "John Doe".

According to the medical examiner, the small cut above his eye, close to the temple, was a stab wound; the blade had broken off and was embedded in his brain. The vomiting was not caused by alcohol, but by increased intracranial pressure and bleeding. Had we taken the time to assess the wound and sent him for a head x-ray, it may have saved his life. Instead, we ignored the obvious symptoms of a head injury and let him sleep it off to eternal rest. The individual who stabbed our patient was found, arrested, and brought to trial. Some lessons are hard to forget.

On the afternoon shift after 7 PM, moonlighting residents from a variety of specialties staff the emergency room. When things were quiet our moonlighting residents would retreat to the sleeping area. We could awaken them to see patients. Being an experienced ER nurse, I assessed the patient and sent the patient for an x-ray, ordered some routine labs, and had everything ready with the results for the resident. I woke them up so they could treat the patient. This expedited things especially late in the evening or during the night. Occasionally, additional blood work or medications were ordered, and as a team, we worked together well. I would leave the emergency room, make my rounds, and return since ER was usually the busiest place in the hospital.

"No, Your Sore Throat for 3 Months Does Not Constitute an Emergency at 2 AM"

One evening I had worked a double shift- my afternoon supervision and the night shift in the emergency department. Occasionally, we saw patients who were not considered a life-and-death emergency. However, some patients had different definitions of an emergency. That night a gentleman showed up at 2 AM and demanded to be seen immediately. It was a quiet night; the physician was soundly asleep. I asked the patient what the problem was. He had a sore throat for 3 months, and this specific night he couldn't stand it any longer. He had no temperature and otherwise seemed okay. I explained to him that this was not a life-and-death matter, like a stroke or heart attack or car accident. "Why have you not seen your private physician for three months?" I just didn't get around to it. Tonight, my throat is terrible." The ER physician saw him, gave him antibiotics, and sent home. The physician was less than cheerful in treating the gentleman and repeated the definition of any emergency. The patient thanked us for the care, felt somewhat embarrassed and left the emergency room with a prescription in hand.

Another unusual nonemergent situation came about when a dad brought in his 2-year-old son who was totally blue. Not cyanotic from head to toe, but blue like a Smurf. His father was painting and was acting as a babysitter while mom ran to the store to get milk. While daddy may have been a good painter, he was not a great babysitter. This cute little African American 2-year-old painted himself blue, from head to toe. He did an excellent job. Dad was concerned that when mom came home and found out, she would kill him. Some of us wondered if that would be considered justifiable homicide.

The hard part was removing the paint. This was oil-based and was very difficult to remove without turning the poor little darling a gorgeous shade of dusty gray. I did my best to remove the paint with a lot of paint thinner, mineral oil, baby oil, anything I could find that worked. He came out looking a little ashen in spots but not too bad. I didn't think his son would be helping him paint in the future. I also didn't think he would be doing much babysitting under the circumstances, if his wife didn't kill him.

One woman who was having a particularly bad day, decided to take a warm bath and soak her troubles away. As she was lying in the tub, she used her big toe to play with a drop of water in the faucet. Eventually, she pushed her toe in deeper, and it got stuck in the faucet. She called her husband, who came in and assessed the situation and decided he was going to get a saw and remove the faucet since he really couldn't unscrew it. The toe was stuck, and no matter what they tried, it was not coming out. On his way to retrieve the saw, he decided that maybe he should just call the fire department, so, he did.

The next thing the wife knew, there were four handsome young men staring at her, naked, in the bathtub. She grabbed the shower curtain and pulled it down to cover herself and then realized it was a clear plastic shower curtain. Not much help there! She was screaming at her husband, "What were you thinking?" The fire department personnel proceeded to saw off the faucet, and she was delivered to the ER, still screaming at her husband, and wrapped in a large bath towel. Once we gave her medication to calm her down, we were able to grease the toe up and slowly slide it out of the faucet. The x-rays showed no damage to the toe, only to the lady's dignity.

One shift a mom came in with her 6-year-old son, who had a small laceration. It did not look like it was anything to get excited about. However, the mother was borderline hysterical and demanded to be seen immediately. I explained to her that we had more critical patients and that her son's laceration did not look that serious. Therefore, she would have to wait. She said, "No, you don't understand. That wasn't the issue. I had put this bleach on my hair and thought I would have time to remove it. If I don't get it off immediately, my hair will fall out."

As a woman, that situation I could understand. I took the mom back and stuck her head over the sink, where I could thoroughly rinse it. She was extremely grateful I saved her hair. It took a while before her son was taken into the emergency room for treatment. It turned out to be a small cut that didn't require stitches. Both were relieved and left the emergency room in better condition than when they arrived. That's always my intent.

What Is That Weird Sound?

Some emergencies are awkward, and patients don't always want to be forthcoming with what's wrong and how it happened. In one situation, the patient arrived with symptoms of G.I. discomfort. That's all he would tell me and wanted to see the doctor. He had a weird noise that emitted from somewhere in his anatomy. I could not figure out the sound. I thought possibly he had an implant of some sort.

The doctor and I were at the bedside to examine this patient. The patient didn't want to say too much in front of me. The doctor tried to subtly signal me to leave. I was dense and didn't get it. So, I asked, "What is that weird sound?" The patient had a vibrator stuck in his rectum; the doctor was a concerned that the battery might leak and kill him. I left the room. The surgeon was able to remove it without any additional concerns.

Some emergencies that are so bizarre they cannot be explained. A blind gentlemen, Mr. Pasquale, came with his daughter to the emergency room complaining of chest pains. Mr. Pasquale lived with his daughter, who was taking care of him for many years. Complaining of chest pains, he presented with typical cardiac symptoms. We started CRP when he went into cardiac arrest. His monitor showed a ventricular fibrillation pattern (life-threatening arrhythmia), so I placed the pads on his chest and the physician was ready to deliver the shock. Just then, Mr. Pasquale raised his hands and grabbed the physician's hands as if to stop him. This was bizarre since the man was in a pattern that was not compatible with life.

When he recovered consciousness, Mr. Pasquale said he saw the expression on the physician's face who was trying to save him, and yet the patient knew he was interfering with the process. He described one of our nurses in the room who had flaming red hair. He later told us that perhaps he was conflicted about whether it was okay to die. He didn't want to leave his family; he just wasn't ready. His daughter and family were grateful that we saved Mr. Pasquale. He recovered in our intensive care unit and eventually went home.

It was a policy in the emergency room that if a mother came to ER in labor, she had to be taken to the OB department by a registered nurse. The reason for it came to light one evening when a pregnant mom showed up with two small boys and four bags full of groceries. It was winter; it was cold, and she had boots on. She told the receptionist that she was in active labor and didn't think she would make it home to put the groceries away and leave the boys with her mother. The boys were well behaved and sat in the emergency room waiting area with the groceries, under the watchful eye of our receptionist.

I took the mom to OB. I brought her to the room, and before she could undress, she fainted across the bed. She still had her boots on, and I tried to get her pants down, but the boots were interfering. I could see she was crowning. I bent over to take a closer look. Just as I did, her water broke, all over my nursing cap, hair, and face. This was her 13th baby. The baby came out shortly after that. Stuff was hanging off my nursing cap. I vowed the next time I would not look that closely! I returned to the emergency room after I washed my hair and, announced she had another boy. She was well underway to having her own basketball team. The brothers were pleased the baby wasn't a girl. They had another playmate, and Mom had more hand-me-downs as well. I wonder if they charged her for the delivery. I wanted my cut if they did!

The Horrors of ER

Anyone who has ever had children can tell you that toddlers can be frustrating. A young mother carried her screaming toddler to the emergency room. The child had severe burns on both hands. However, this was no accident. The young mom, fearing she was losing her battle with potty training, placed her motherly love on the back burner and her toddler' s hands on the front burner causing 2nd and 3rd degree burns to the palms of the hands and fingers. It was hard to forget those screams! The burns would heal after a lot of painful interventions and physical therapy. The mental wounds caused by the only person this toddler unconditionally loved may never heal. Child Protective Services removed the child from home and the police arrested her. As nurses, we all felt this mother needed coping and parenting skills rather than jail time, not the best environment for learning those skills.

The Dead Baby

This incident was relayed to me by a very experienced ER nurse who was extremely distraught. It was late in the evening when this male, appearing to be in his mid-40s, presented to the emergency room wearing a trench coat wrapped around his protruding abdomen. To the horror of the emergency room staff when the trench coat was removed, the patient presented with a dead 5 to 6-month-old baby stuck on his erected penis. According to the patient he attempted to have sex with the baby and, in so doing, smothered the infant. Police were immediately notified; They placed the patient under arrest after he was treated. Just when you think you've seen it all, man's atrocity, depravity, or insanity presents itself.

No Rest for The Weary!

Besides patients and families, we also dealt with some of the challenging personalities of our moonlighting residents. Dr. Bannon comes to mind, who was less than thrilled to work when he was on duty. After all, he had already put in a full day as a resident and was looking forward to a quiet shift in the middle of the week. As anyone whoever has worked the ER knows, shifts are never predictable. There are rarely quiet evenings in the ER. I could sometimes predict our busy times, like after church on Sundays, after Kmart closed most nights, or when dad came home from work and mom could take the kids to the ER.

This specific night was extremely busy. To keep Dr. Bannon happy, we would hide the charts. Just as he finished one case, we produced another patient to be seen. He eventually looked at the time, when the patient was originally written up, and our plan fell apart. But it was good while it lasted.

I was amazed with the effectiveness of the teamwork in the ER and how everybody anticipated the needs of the patients, the families, and our physicians to keep things moving smoothly. Emergency room work is not for everybody. It's one of those areas where you have to think fast on your feet, prioritize, and act promptly. You need to anticipate the patient's needs.

There are no egos in an ER, or at least there shouldn't be. Everybody is there to do a job, no matter how small, it mattered. That's why I found it challenging and rewarding. I saw l lots of opportunities to educate patients and families to keep them from making return visits. If you visited an ER today, you may or may not be seen by a physician. You may be seen and treated by a physicians' assistant, or an advanced practice nurse. Your presenting problem may be the only thing looked at and treated, with no consideration for comorbidities like high blood pressure, diabetes, which may have led to your chief complaint and reason for the emergency room visit. Years ago, I was able to take the time to look at the whole patient with all their problems and educate them where I could.

After many years of working the afternoon and midnight shift, I was considering finding in nursing position on the day shift. This transition would allow me to spend more time in the evening with my family. I was ready to explore a different avenue of nursing.

CHAPTER ELEVEN

FLIGHT **N**URSING **101**

*"Just be prepared for a long and
often uncertain journey. The good
stuff doesn't come easy."*

—Tim Westergren

INTO THE **W**ILD **B**LUE **Y**ONDER

REMEMBER **E**LAINE **FROM** Chapter One? She wasn't the only one who influenced my career. Elaine married her high school sweetheart, Bill Boyke, who served his country as a captain in the US Air Force. He was so handsome in his blue uniform, which perfectly matched Elaine's blue cape. They were an awesome couple.

While in high school, I expressed my interest in serving my country at some point as a dedicated nurse caring for wounded soldiers. Bill suggested

I join the Civil Air Patrol. This is an organization formed shortly after the attack on Pearl Harbor. Volunteer small aircraft pilots assisted in search and rescue missions for downed aircraft. That sounded like fun. My dad, who had military experience, was less than thrilled with the thought of his daughter going into military service.

When I joined the Civil Air Patrol, I learned about aeronautics, the principles of flight, and search and rescue missions. We had mock search and rescue exercises, where we practiced those observation skills. As a nurse, you can never learn too much about observation skills. It was an excellent experience. Later, I developed an interest in getting a private pilot's license and possibly getting more involved at a senior level with the Civil Air Patrol. I spent many enjoyable years with the Civil Air Patrol. I participated in some search and rescue missions as my busy nursing and family work schedule allowed.

A navy man, my husband always dreamed of being a top gun aviator. That was impossible due to his eyesight, but he still was fascinated with aviation. We both decided to pursue private pilot's licenses. We finished the program, were cleared by FAA, and could now take off into the wild blue yonder pursuing yet another adventure.

After becoming a private pilot, I often took my son Ryan flying with me on short runs hoping he would enjoy aviation as much as I did. One time, I spoke with a group who landed at the city airport. They needed a motel in which to spend the night. While our conversation continued, I turned around and noticed my son was missing. I couldn't imagine where he went. To my surprise, he took the clipboard and keys to a Piper Tomahawk and went out on the tarmac to check the plane out for flight. He was ready to go, but I wasn't. When I noticed the keys missing, I frantically ran out to the plane. While I was taking my flying lessons, Ryan sat in the office, watching all the videos on how to fly a plane. (He got a pilot's license at a much older age.) Ryan had watched me do a "go around" and prepare the plane for flight. He was at the aircraft, and I questioned the security guard how Ryan entered the tarmac without an adult. His response was, "He said you were going to go fly, and he went ahead to get the plane ready." I was not impressed with that rationale considering Ryan was about six-years-old at the time. I asked Ryan how to start the plane. He explained in detail exactly how the process went. Now I was concerned! I can only imagine him getting into the plane, starting it, and taking off. That may have been the start of my grey hair.

My pilot's license was rated for visual-flight rules (VFR), allowing me to fly if the weather permitted me to see the ground clearly. The next step would be the instrument-rated flight rules (IFR) that allowed for the use of instruments when ground visibility was impossible. I did not want to train for that; for me, IFR meant "I follow roads", which is exactly what I did.

I shared the skies with the best of them. There's nothing like the freedom of flying high in the sky and looking down at the earth. My flight instructor once asked me how I felt about flying. I told him that it was so quiet and peaceful; I thought you could reach out and touch the face of God. He reminded me that I was a lot closer to God in my landings than I ever was in flying.

On one close call, I lost an engine on takeoff from City Airport in Detroit. I managed to get composed, restart the engine, and keep flying. The control tower asked me if I wanted to return. I said, "No, thank you. I want to get high up and far away, compose myself, and then come home."

Terror in the Sky

Since a few pilots at the airport knew that I was also a nurse, one of them approached me with an opportunity to escort a patient from Florida in a private jet back to the Metropolitan Medical

Center for treatment. It sounded like a perfect job for me. I was excited, and as a nurse, I would be the only one taking care of the patient and saving his life. As a bonus, if something inadvertently happened to the pilot, I could also take over and fly the plane to safety. Who was I kidding? I was terrified. I knew when the wheels fold up in a plane, you have no backup. The plane can't pull over the side of the road and wait for an ambulance to show up. I quickly decided to subdue my anxiety; the patient's life depended on me. Now there's a sobering thought.

Fortunately, the patient, who suffered a mild stroke, had stable vital signs, and slept the whole flight. His wife, on the other hand, was a basket case. She had never flown in anything smaller than a 747. We were in a nicely equipped, expensive Learjet. She was not impressed. I assured her that we would get her and her husband home safely. She was not that convinced and asked, "If there's a problem, what should I do?" I simply told her, "Just follow my directions, and we will be fine." (I had no idea what I would do if there were a problem.)

Just for curiosity's sake, I went into the cockpit to talk to the pilot and see what's happening. What I saw cured my constipation! The entire window they were looking out to fly the plane was utterly iced and frosted over. We were at an altitude of 40,000 feet, just above commercial airlines. I knew the temperature decreases with every 1000 feet of altitude. When I returned to my seat, I looked at the window next to me and saw a trickle of water rolling down. I could see a little bit of a concerning look on his wife's face, so I just calmly reached over and pulled down the shade. That's when I decided to return to the cockpit to let the pilot know and see what's going on.

To my shock, I saw the pilot using his oxygen mask; he had an unusual bluish/gray color to his face. I asked the copilot, "Is he OK? Does he do this often?" The copilot assured me that he's fine, and the pilot gave me a thumbs up. I sincerely hope they weren't kidding because I didn't have a clue how to fly a jet.

We landed safely; an ambulance met us to whisk the patient and his wife to Metropolitan Medical Center for treatment. I was greatly relieved to give up that adventure and keep my feet on the ground. Unfortunately, several months later, I heard the plane I flew in crashed. The pilot and co-pilot were both killed. I guess it wasn't my turn to leave the planet! That was sobering news.

I wanted more information about flight nursing, so I joined the ASHBEAMS (American Society of

Hospital-Based Emergency Air Medical Services). Established in 1989, this organization of flight nurses fly in a helicopter or fixed-wing aircraft to transport patients or as part of an organ donor team. While attending one of their conferences in Denver, I heard two of the helicopters crashed with all occupants killed. I had to rethink my interest in flight nursing as a career; I had too much to live for.

At least I had a successful experience. Like any specialty within nursing or any profession for that matter, explore the pros and cons before committing. For me, turning my back on flight nursing was best to keep both feet on the ground.

CHAPTER TWELVE

SPORTS MEDICINE-PLAYING WITH THE BIG BOYS

"The quality of a person's life is in direct proportion to their commitment to excellence, regardless of their chosen field of endeavor."

— Vince Lombardi

IT WAS TIME for me to explore my options in nursing care delivery on the day shift. Our son, Ryan, was born in January that year and I wanted to spend my evenings with my husband and family. I fell back on my experiences in orthopedics and decided to take a position as nurse manager of Sports Medicine and Joint Replacement at Townsend Hospital, part of the Metropolitan Medical Center. As the nurse manager, I was responsible for the care delivered to famous and infamous sports figures, as well as individuals requiring joint replacement who were admitted to my nursing unit.

My first encounter with Townsend Hospital was as a student nurse. I worked weekends in the nursing office as a receptionist. I typed seven copies of the operating room (OR) schedule for Monday morning and distributed them to the nursing units.

This job took place before computers allowed you to hit the button and send the document to print. I had to make seven carbon copies on an electric type-writer. If you made a mistake, you made it through seven sheets, erasing, and re-typing. Anyone can tell you I am not a typist. I use the Columbus method: I discover, then land. It may not sound practical, but it did get me through two master's degrees, looking at the keyboard while typing.

It took me a long time to type the OR schedule if I was uninterrupted. I was never uninterrupted. Several people would stop by the nursing office— residents, and other nurses— just to chat. I heard a lot of exciting stories and got skilled in people and time management by the time I was finished. Those were valuable skills in my future.

The Chief of Sports Medicine was Dr. Brian MacDonald, better known to all of us as the "knee god". Dr. MacDonald took care of several professional Detroit-based sports teams such as the Detroit Red Wings, our hockey team, and Detroit Pistons, our basketball team. He worked with various other athletes who showed up on my doorstep.

We nurses met once a week with Dr. MacDonald, residents, and the OR team. The discussion focused on patients who might present various challenges to care. Occasionally we discussed the surgical procedures and a variety of assessment techniques. The nurses on this unit were exceptionally trained. When they called a physician with an assessment of "anterior drawer sign" (a test to determine the stability of the anterior cruciate ligament of the knee), the physician knew the assessment was probably accurate.

How to Hide Famous People on a Small Nursing Unit

It was interesting to try to hide one of the celebrities when they came in for a procedure. I would often find some of the women from the business office showing up in high heels and scrubs to just walk by the unit in the hope of getting a peek at our celebrities. There was a dry erase board that listed the patient's name, room number, and attending physician. The challenge became to hide the celebrity by changing their names, room numbers, and occasionally their sex. It was always fascinating to watch people slowly and casually stroll through the unit with the pretense of dropping off some papers or getting information. I became successful at hiding them. I believe the patients had a right to privacy regardless of their social or athletic status.

One year, Detroit had a rough hockey season. Almost every player came to us for repairs. One such player was "Sam" (I gave him that name to protect his identity and possibly his dignity). Sam was quite a lady's man. At the time, my 13 year-old daughter, Hollie, was working as a candy striper on my unit. She was exploring the possibility of choosing nursing as a career. Hollie would deliver fresh water, run errands for the nursing staff, and generally visit with the patients to cheer them up. Hollie had flowing curly dark hair; Sam was quite interested in frequently seeing her. One of my nursing assistants mentioned to me that Sam might be getting a little too friendly with Hollie. I mentioned to Sam that Hollie was my daughter. He replied, "She is really beautiful; I'd like to date her." I said, "That would be nice in maybe 10-15 years from now, but she's only 13". He continued to refer to her as "jailbait" and suggested, rather than trying to hide the celebrities on the floor, to hide her. He was nice enough to sign a team photo for her, which she has today.

The physician of one of the hockey players from the opposing team admitted him for a broken wrist one night. I took care of his wrist and made him comfortable. While in the hospital, he learned his new team would be the Detroit Red Wings, who were the ones who broke his wrist. I felt sorry for him. He was on the phone with his family – his mother and his girlfriend, who lived in Montreal. His biggest complaint was that quite often, professional players were a commodity and traded literally without their knowledge. If you want to play the game, you play the game *well*. We all made him feel at home, the best we could under the circumstances. In caring for these athletes, we realized the fans often do not understand or appreciate the sacrifices the athletes and their families make for the sake of the sport.

Our customers did not consist of just local talent. One of our patients was a young, extremely tall 7-foot 2 inches basketball player from Italy. He spoke very little English, so I used a lot of sign language that was generally effective. He came in the day before his surgery and completed all the paperwork with the help of an interpreter.

The next morning, getting him ready for surgery was a bit of a challenge due to the language barrier and his being unfamiliar with hospital routines. I gave him a hospital gown, and the perplexed look on his face told me he needed a demonstration on how this worked. I showed him that it tied in the back, and he nodded that he understood. Within a few minutes, he appeared in the hallway outside his room wearing the hospital gown. It covered this tall man to just a little below his chest. I ran to preserve his modesty and wrapped a sheet like a skirt around his waist; he was embarrassed but didn't know what else to do. The player had a successful surgical outcome and was soon on his way to recovery to play basketball in Italy.

 We often had to scramble to find interpreters for some of our celebrity athletes who arrived from foreign countries. This was just another one of those exciting challenges in nursing.

One famous basketball player came in for hand surgery. The OR sterilized a basketball to make sure after the repair, he could still wrap his fingers around a basketball. His career depended on it. For that matter, the surgeon's reputation depended on it as well. All turned out well, and he continued to play basketball and created quite a name for himself.

They May Look Tough, But I Can Scare Them

My unit also took care of football players. One man I cared for was huge. He was a tough-look-ing guy, with lots of muscles. As big and tough as he was, he was terrified of an IV. I had a way of calming down the big boys or scaring them by reminding them that I controlled their pain meds. They were on my turf now, and the expectations were a little different. They now had to play by my rules. My job was to safely deliver them to the OR and to take care of the postoperative needs until they left to get injured again, which most of them did. They were always welcome back.

IF IT NO LONGER WORKS, WE'LL GIVE YOU A NEW ONE

Another interesting population on the unit was our joint replacement patients. That segment of orthopedics was under the direction of Dr. Gary Keifer, an excellent, focused surgeon with just a touch of OCD (obsessive-compulsive disorder). Dr. Keifer was never one minute early or one minute late for rounds on his patients. You could set your watch by his punctuality.

A warm and fuzzy bedside manner, however, was not one of his strong points. A retired English schoolteacher who had a hip replacement was articulate in describing Dr. Keifer's lack of a pleasant bedside manner. She told him he did not know how to speak English. Instead, he spoke medical gibberish to his patients. That did not put him in a good mood when dealing with the nursing staff.

Dr. Keifer took on one of our nurses, who we referred to as "Princess" due to her personality traits. When he loudly and publicly chastised her, she remained calm and picked up the phone to page "Code 69." We called a Code 69 whenever a physician yelled at a nurse. Any available nurse arrived and surrounded the victim as a show of support. When Dr. Keifer turned around and saw approximately 20 nurses staring at him, he decided it was much wiser just to leave the unit. As nurse manager, I dealt with the aftermath of this all too frequent encounter.

Mr. Brown was another one of my more memorable patients. He was approximately 6 foot 6, a former heavyweight boxer with a bad limp from a deteriorating hip. Mr. Brown was a soft-spoken but a scary-looking individual. The prosthetic needed to be custom designed because of his weight and height. The artificial hip was made of stainless steel, weighed several pounds, and was greater than 12 inches long.

Dr. Keifer made postoperative rounds with his physician assistant (PA) at exactly 8 AM. The physician assistant was the only person who changed postoperative dressings. I questioned why Dr. Keifer did not allow the nursing staff to change postoperative dressings since this is a common practice in nursing. Dr. Keifer advised me he didn't trust the nurses' knowledge base, but his PA knew exactly what and how he wanted things done. (Remember his OCD!)

Unfortunately, the PA was not available on the weekends; therefore, Mr. Brown's dressing was not changed. Monday morning, I arrived early on the unit to make my rounds before the surgical team rounds. I went into Mr. Brown's room and noticed a heavy order emitting from the surgical site dressing. I pulled back the surgical dressing; it looked like a green surgical towel. The wound was infected with a pseudomonas bacterium (which has a peculiar odor and green drainage).

 I immediately changed the dressing, placed it in a plastic bag, cleaned the wound, obtained a culture, and applied a new sterile dressing. When Dr. Keifer made rounds, he commented the patient was doing well, and the dressing looked fine. I informed him the dressing looked fine because I just changed it, since his PA was not available, and showed him the plastic bag containing the green soaked old dressing. "The nursing staff is available 24/7 for any patient care needs, such as sterile dressing changes. You can depend on the nurses to follow any specific instructions you might have for dressing changes." After seeing the dressing, Dr. Keifer agreed. The physician ordered antibiotics; Mr. Brown recovered quite well from his surgery.

There were a lot of changes taking place in the Metropolitan Medical Center. I heard of a plan in place to merge several hospitals under the umbrella of the Metropolitan Medical Center, giving more buying power to the organization as well as the ability to share expensive equipment. The Finance Department put the plan together based on the cost of doing business but did not take a lot of consideration in how the physicians, who bring in the business, would react. Each hospital would have designated specific specialties. At that time, each hospital had its separate chief of specialty services, such as orthopedics, oncology, pediatrics, etc. Relocating the specialties to a designated hospital, and not duplicating specialties in each hospital, meant the loss of that status of "the chief of ..." for a lot of physicians. They were not happy, probably because they were not consulted. That disgruntled physicians' meeting took place on my unit. I didn't know if I should serve cookies and coffee or something much stronger! Everybody had an opinion, but it didn't matter. The Finance Department's decisions took effect.

An opportunity soon emerged for me to take a position in a hospital much closer to my home. The position was a lateral move to the role of clinical manager for orthopedics. At the time, and with all the uncertainty regarding whether my unit would remain or be dispersed, it looked like a good idea to take advantage of this opportunity.

CHAPTER THIRTEEN

PLAYING WITH THE REALLY BIG BOYS

*"If it doesn't challenge you,
it doesn't change you"*

—Anonymous

MY NEW POSITION was manager for an orthopedic unit at Bonaventure Hospital. The orthopedic unit at Bonaventure Hospital was quite different from the Sports Medicine and Joint Replacement unit at Townsend Hospital in the Metropolitan Medical Center. At Bonaventure, I had a staff of approximately 75 nurses to care for a unit of 40 beds. There were only 2 LPNs; this was an almost all RN staff, which was unusual. Other hospitals staffed nursing units with nurses' aides and LPN's for the majority of the patient care but not Bonaventure Hospital. The average patient assignment on the day shift was 4 to 5 patients. This was about half of what it was at the Metropolitan Medical Center.

The workload as manager of orthopedics wasn't any different than it was working at Townsend Hospital, except for having a large RN nursing staff. We had about 12 orthopedic surgeons at the time, who had an excellent professional working relationship with the nursing staff. Although the nursing care provided was outstanding, it did not meet the higher clinical expertise of the Townsend nurses.

It was, at times, challenging to get the nurses to work together. Some helped only their friends. It was soon apparent I had to come up with a plan to make everyone feel needed, valued, and encouraged to share in the workload for the sake of the patient.

One of the methods that worked for me was a "bring your best dish" potluck lunch. The only restriction was that they could talk about anything *except* work. As the nurses got to know each other and to appreciate their personal lives, they began to empathize and work with each other as team members.

- The staff learned Sarah took care of her husband (who had a stroke) before she came to work. They realized this could be why she was tired all the time and not ready to jump in and help her coworkers when the need arose.

- Sheila had multiple sclerosis. Her symptoms were not obvious most of the time, and she did what she could, but there were days where there wasn't a lot she could handle.

- Another nurse, Pat, worked the afternoon shift. She had three teenagers at home, and that was the reason she was on the phone continually checking up on them while worrying about what they were doing when she wasn't there.

When people started to understand problems, everybody began to share in the workload.

I also created a "brat board" for the staff to post pictures of their children, the reason why they worked so hard. Some posted pets, their furry children, and it was interesting to see how the kids grew from year to year.

The newsletter was my next venture. It listed memos that impacted the work, recipes, jokes, an interesting insight article, and a secret number that was printed somewhere within an article. Whoever was the first to bring me the number won a small prize. If nothing else, it broke up the monotony of a day-to-day routine, and I knew they read it.

The National Association of Orthopedic Nurses offered a certification exam that recognized orthopedic nursing as a specialty. I took the exam and became credentialed as an ONC (Orthopedic Nurse Certified). I felt this was important to add credibility to my position as a manager and to assist in educating my staff.

Our patients were generic orthopedic patients: fractures, joint replacements, multiple skeletal issues, arthritis, and so on. The hospital was not a research facility. We didn't do anything creative; it was basic good orthopedic care. Some of the staff members became credentialed as orthopedic nurses as well, which added to the credibility of the unit. But some problems remained. Now that the nurses worked better together, it was time to get the physicians involved.

I remembered Dr. MacDonald's Monday morning team meetings, addressing upcoming patients, and improving assessment skills. I envisioned "lunch and learn sessions" with the orthopedic doctors. I approached the few who I felt comfortable with; they were willing to discuss some of the upcoming cases as well as bring some unusual X-Rays. They also shared some information about the type of patients they saw in their practice. These sessions educated the nursing staff on the complex world of orthopedics and gave a lot of credibility to the unit. Also, the nurses felt they were part of a team, not just following doctors' orders and completing tasks.

The hospital didn't have orthopedic residents per se but had family practice residents who were welcome to join in on our sessions. This became quite popular. The doctors sometimes brought in lunch for everybody during our meetings, or some of the staff would bring in their favorites dishes to pass around. I could see camaraderie rebuilding on the unit. This was important to provide the type of care that I had expected from my staff.

Occasionally staffing was an issue. Most of the nurses worked 8-hour shifts: 7:00 AM to 3:00 PM, 3:00 PM to 11:00 PM, and 11:00 PM to 7:00 AM. Few requested 12-hour shifts, and, at the time, it was possible to work them into the schedule. The staff worked every other weekend at Bonaventure Hospital. At Townsend Hospital, they worked two weekends a month, which could be consecutive or not.

When I first started as manager, I put together a schedule based on the needs of the unit. I posted the schedule. When I arrived on Monday morning, there was a lineup of nurses waiting to educate me on how scheduling worked at Bonaventure. Their schedules were literally set in stone; they could tell me what weekend they had to work around a holiday five years in advance. I adjusted the schedule. I got it. To cover gaps in the schedule, I posted a calendar called "Conklin's Crisis Corner", indicating daily what level of help I needed. The staff could sign up for overtime; some were grateful for the opportunity to make a few extra bucks. The unit was now running smoothly.

Bonaventure implemented a service line management program to improve patient care delivery. The hospital administration approached me to take over the Orthopedic Service Line. Now that was a challenge! It involved strategic planning in looking into the future to see what services we could provide, how to make them better, and how to please everybody: the patient, the physician, the departments, and so on. Sure, I can do this, no problem. Little did I know how interesting this would become.

Service Line Management or Lack Thereof

The basic concept of service line management was to group all services impacting a patient under one manager who was empowered to make changes to improve care delivery. I don't know why that sounded so easy. It made a lot of sense. From my perspective, there were a few things that could improve, one of which was getting the patient to and from the physical therapy department.

The Physical Therapy Department (PT) was located on the lower level, and we were on the third floor. To get a patient on time for a physical therapy session, the nurses would get the patient out of bed, call transportation, wait for them to arrive, and deliver the patient to PT. The reverse also happened in physical therapy once a session was finished. They would call for transport to take the patient back to the room. The patient was tired and had to sit in the wheelchair waiting for transportation to arrive.

I thought the physical therapist should be the person getting the patients safely in and out of bed and showing the patient how to ambulate rather than the nurses doing it and then sending them to physical therapy to learn how to do that. As the Orthopedic Service Line Manager, I proposed relocating at least a small portion of physical therapy, like parallel bars and an exercise table, to the nursing unit to avoid some of the confusion with transportation efforts.

The doctors loved the idea. It made sense to have physical therapy on the unit where the physicians can see the patient making some progress. On the other hand, the physical therapy department was not so enthusiastic. However, we are all there for the patient's sake, and soon they decided that this is not such a bad idea after all. The physical therapists created a small area equipped with essential physical therapy paraphernalia. The patients weren't as tired getting to physical therapy and were able to participate better. It was a win-win situation all around.

Another significant issue was that of reimbursement. The Diagnostic Related Groups (DRGs) classified hospital cases into one of the original four hundred and sixty-seven groups. DRG 209 particularly dealt with joint replacement. (DRG 209 has changed over the years and included more specific classifications). On average, patients who had hips or knees replaced stayed at the hospital for *21* days.

At the time I was Orthopedic Service Line Manager, DRG 209 was paying for a length of stay of *10* days. We were losing money with every patient who stayed longer than 10 days. I met with the orthopedic surgeons and shared how our reimbursement issues impacted the bottom line. I encouraged them to tell their patients that they would be in the hospital as long as necessary rather than a blanket three week stay. They were receptive to the idea and encouraged their patients to focus on going home rather than staying in the hospital. That worked! The joint replacement patients were discharged within 14 days. After several months, the length of stay was shortened to 7 to 10 days. This was a reflection on moving physical therapy to the orthopedic unit and allowing patients to participate more without the element of fatigue.

Part of my other responsibility as Orthopedic Service Line Manager was to develop a strategic plan for the next five years, outlining the opportunities I saw could be implemented. I assessed our competition's offerings as it related to orthopedics. One of the suggestions I submitted was the creation of a training sports facility for boys and girls, ages ten through eighteen. This would prevent a lot of injuries to children who did not have a good grasp on body mechanics and at times, were too eager to succeed. The administration agreed with the idea and purchased some equipment. This allowed the orthopedic surgeons to volunteer some of their expertise as well as our physical therapy staff in training children to prevent injuries. The program was quite successful. The Orthopedic Service Line netted the hospital a profit of several million dollars per year.

The senior administration staff noticed my successes. The CEO, Mr. Robert Ellison, asked me to become the director over all the service lines. At the time, Bonaventure Hospital had five service lines: orthopedics, aging services, cardiology, emergency room, and the operating room. Each service line had their own manager scrutinizing the services offered, did strategic planning, and improved services to our patient population. The hospital had a patient satisfaction rating of 98%. This was great for our new concepts.

I was surprised to be asked to take over the endeavor since I did not have a master's degree, and the remainder of the senior administration staff were all vice presidents. I was just a manager and a nurse. I would become part of the senior administration staff. Was I ready for this challenge? Oh, why not, if I can fly a plane and navigate my way around a lot of staffing issues, how hard can this be? I was about to find out.

WORKING WITH A HAMMER AND NO OTHER TOOLS

Our senior administrative management staff consisted of all-male vice presidents of various departments, a nun (representing the order that originally built the hospital), and me. My new position as Director of Service Lines reported directly to the CEO. That was also a challenge. If I were unable to get data from any of the vice presidents in a timely manner, Mr. Ellison would march to their office and demand my needed data by 5 PM. Needless to say, this did not endear me to the other vice presidents. It was like working with only a hammer in the toolbox and no additional tools.

I prevailed and managed to get along with everybody. Mr. Ellison eventually moved on and was replaced by the chief operating officer Mr. Ed Mooney, who did not particularly like me. I doubt if he thought I was a threat to his position. It may have stemmed from a meeting where I gave Mr. Ellison my report for the month, which differed considerably from Mr. Mooney's report on the same topic. The question arose during our meeting about the discrepancy. I could explain my numbers. However, Mr. Mooney had some difficulty explaining his data. It was a rather embarrassing moment for him. But when Mr. Mooney moved into the temporary CEO position, he decided that the Director of Service Lines should have a master's degree. My position disappeared, and he replaced me with someone who had a master's degree.

I missed my hands-on patient care. Even as the orthopedic service line manager, I would often show up on the orthopedic unit, adjusting slings and traction. My staff very politely invited me to leave and let them take care of the patients. I didn't take it personally; they knew I enjoyed working with the patients, and I knew my staff was better trained.

My replacement on the orthopedic unit as manager had a somewhat warped sense of humor. She asked me one day to remove a drain from a patient. She hadn't done this before and did not feel comfortable. I told her I would be glad to help her and would take her with me to show her how it's done. After I pulled the drain, she looked at me and stated, "I think that was the right patient." My heart sunk to my shoes since the attending orthopedic surgeon had a personality of fireworks and was not afraid to go off at any given moment. I immediately checked the chart for the order, which I should've done in the first place, to find this was the correct patient, and everything was fine. Another important lesson learned: verify, verify, verify.

When my position closed, I was offered a staff position. While I enjoyed patient care, I learned so much in management and wanted to continue in that role if possible or explore an area of nursing that was challenging. It was time to make that decision. I evaluated the opportunities in the Metropolitan Medical Center. I noted a position opening in the spinal cord intensive care unit where I could use my orthopedic background. This looked promising. Another challenge awaits!

Within a few short months, I completed my studies and received my master of science degree in administration with a focus on healthcare administration. Interesingly, my master thesis dealt with the challenges of a service line concept. I had a lot of experience with those challenges and was able to overcome some of the road blocks and make a difference. I was ready to take some of those skills and apply them to my next adventure.

CHAPTER FOURTEEN

JOINING THE ELITE NURSES OF THE ICU

"Great nurses are levelheaded during times of crisis. In critical care, crisis is an everyday occurrence but the levelheaded nurse stays calm, looks at the whole picture and gets to work."

—Michelle Post, RN, BSN, SCRN

...AND I THOUGHT I KNEW A LOT

THE NURSING ADMINISTRATION of City Receiving Hospital, a Level I trauma center and part of the Metropolitan Medical Center, offered me a position in the Spinal Cord Intensive Care Unit. Although Orthopedics was my passion, working with spinal cord injured patients was a challenge. Intensive care nursing was quite different than nursing on the medical surgical units. In the critical care unit,

I had one patient, possibly two, and I got to know the patients, their medical histories, and relatives.

My orientation consisted of several weeks of classroom instruction on various aspects of intensive care nursing, assessment, additional equipment, and calculation of the numerous IV medications that sustained life and blood pressures. I found the concepts difficult but was up for the challenge. I wanted to expand my horizons in nursing. By that time, my master's degree seemed to intimidate my first preceptor. I don't know why. I certainly had a lot to learn, and she had a lot to teach me. The nurse manager assigned me a different preceptor who was not intimidated by my knowledge.

The Spinal Intensive Care Unit had 12-hour shifts, and I chose the 7 PM to 7 AM shift due to family needs and my belief that it was generally a little less hectic on nights. So I thought; I was quite wrong. The 7 PM to 7 PM shift is generally the one that gets all the trauma cases who show up from the ER or the repeat surgical patients.

To clear a misconception, patients do not sleep all night unless they are in a coma. The majority of my patients were still under anesthesia, so I had a lot to do for them. In the critical care unit, vital signs aren't taken every couple of hours, they are taken every *hour*, or sometimes every half hour, or every 15 minutes, depending on the need. When I say it's intensive care, I do mean intensive care; I watched them like a hawk.

My new preceptor, Kathy, who was usually the charge nurse, was phenomenal. She could run circles around any of the residents dealing with spinal cord injury. Not only could she assess the patient faster from head to toe, but she could also tell you what lab values affected what. Kathy was quite willing to teach. She laughed a lot at me. She was unintimidated by my master's degree, knew a lot, taught a lot, and loved her patients.

In addition to the spinal cord trauma patients, I cared for people with head trauma. Most of the injuries stemmed from either car accidents, gunshot wounds, or blunt trauma from baseball bats, and so on.

We continuously monitored these patients for increased intracranial pressures, which at times would send them back to the OR. Some of the cases were just unbelievable. One very drunk individual and his buddy, equally drunk, took turns hitting themselves on the head with a baseball bat to see who was the last one standing. My patient lost the bet and almost his life due to massive blunt force head trauma.

City Receiving Hospital soon opened a head trauma unit. To the relief of my staff, those patients were transferred to that area rather than mixing them with the spinal cord population.

One summer, we had so many teenagers the hospital decided to make a small video with the theme being "watch who you hang around with". This started when two boys (ages 14 and 16) were at a party. One of the boys fell asleep on a couch. He was struck by a bullet from a drive-by shooter, making him a paraplegic. He was an innocent kid taking a nap. There were so many of these stories. Our local TV news channel showed the clip; we rented it out to anyone who had teenagers and wanted to view the video.

One tragic incident involved a woman who had twin boys. They were both in their late 20s when they attended a cousin's birthday party. Both of her sons were well educated. One was an accountant, and the other one was working on an advanced college degree. Both were married and had children. While at the cousin's birthday party, the boys were shot when an argument arose between some of the guests. When the men arrived in our unit, one was a paraplegic. The other son was in much more severe condition and was not expected to live.

The mother sat at the bedside, not saying a word. She stared into space. When I talked to her, she gave one-word responses. At the time one of her sons died, the other one was still in a coma. I watched her reaction: she didn't say anything. She looked like she just accepted the fact.

This wasn't a normal reaction. I thought she should be at least crying or something showing some emotion. I put my arm around her and said, "A mother should never have to bury her children." That opened the floodgates. She grabbed me, and we both wept. As a single mother, she raised two successful sons who married, had families, and good jobs. Now she was left with one son who would be in a wheelchair for the rest of his life if he survived, and one who died. She believed her efforts in raising them was a waste of time. I felt sorry for her and for the many families who we dealt with over the years with tragic endings, mostly due to poor choices or just simply being in the wrong place at the wrong time.

Another sad case was a young woman in her 20s who was diagnosed with HIV. She decided she was going to commit suicide by driving her car at 100 miles an hour into a tree. She did not die; instead, she suffered severe head and spinal cord injuries. She was barely alive when she was brought to the unit.

An older gentleman came with her. I needed admission papers signed, but he said he was not her father. He explained that he found her as a baby when he worked for the gas company. While making a call in a house, he discovered a prostitute in bed with her customer, and a crying baby was on the floor in the corner. The gas company employee asked her, "Aren't you going to do anything about your baby?" She said, "You want it, take it", so he did. He brought the baby home, and he and his wife raised her like their own daughter.

Now we had a legal issue in the critical care unit because we couldn't treat her without the consent of her mother. Social Services intervened, and the matter was resolved. Despite our best efforts, she did not survive her serious injuries.

The one thing I did not have to worry about in the spinal cord unit was our patients getting out of bed and walking away or getting lost. Nobody moved. We had some special beds that accommodated patients to prevent complications such as pneumonia, pressure ulcers, and so on. The most frequently used bed was the ROTO bed. It had 4-inch foam pads, in three sections, providing the needed support and alignment. The patient was strapped in, including a head support, to prevent any misalignment of the spine and to secure the patient to the bed. The bed rotated side to side to prevent pulmonary and pressure ulcer issues.

Kathy thought that since I was new, I should experience what it's like to be a patient in a ROTO bed. This bed rotates 180 degrees from one side all the way to the other side. The rotation takes approximately five minutes to complete. Some patients loved it because they felt it was rocking them to sleep. Others were terrified, especially if their injury resulted from a fall. They woke up as the bed was rotating, giving them the sensation they were falling again. Imagine opening your eyes and seeing the walls coming down. We always had a few screams to address during the night.

All the cushions were so secure the patients felt like they were being hugged. Some became dizzy from the rotation; we alleviated that sensation with medication.

I took Kathy's advice and crawled into a ROTO bed that we had ready for a patient. Kathy strapped me in just like you would a patient, with the side packs up against the body, locked in position, and placed straps across my knees so they wouldn't bend. She then started the rotation so I would have an idea of what it felt like. It's a little claustrophobic, but it wasn't too bad. When I asked her to get me out of it, she said "okay" and left the room. Here I was, trapped and tied down, with work to do. I called her name, and she simply replied, "Relax, get used to it." Just at that time, the nursing supervisor was making rounds and wanted to know who the new noisy patient was. Kathy simply told her, "She's just not happy to be here; she's just new." Without looking at me, the supervisor continued her rounds and left. Kathy eventually let me escape. I realized that while the ROTO bed was relatively comfortable, you can't move a muscle. It is quite secure.

Some of our cases had positive endings. Pablo was a 17 or 18-year old teenager who was headed for gang membership. He was in a car accident in which the seat belt did not catch. He struck his knees on the dashboard, causing a paraplegic spinal cord injury.

Pablo was such a lady's man. He had a line that would melt butter. Despite his injuries, he was not bitter. He said, "This is the greatest thing that happened to me because I would not make it to age 30 in a gang". He collected several million dollars from the auto industry and was able to put his older brother in business. Because Michigan has a "no fault" auto insurance, the settlement enabled him to remodel his home to include a new kitchen, ramps for easy access to the home, and special appliances to allow for safe cooking from a wheelchair. He was able to build an addition on the house to accommodate his parents moving in with him. Pablo had many friends visiting him, mostly female. They all felt so sorry for him, and he played that tune very well.

Every year the Spinal Cord Unit had a picnic when we invited our former patients and families to see how everybody was doing. Pablo was always the first to arrive with the stories and jokes. He was such a pleasure to be around despite his injuries.

A lot of our patients' marriages fell apart because of this type of catastrophic injury. Often parents who had finally seen their children become independent pre-accident realized they were coming back home for complete 24/7 care. This was difficult for everybody. Some progressed to being semi-independent, while others totally gave up but just wanted to die.

For example, we took care of Evan. Evan's wife kept nagging him to clean the gutters. It had rained; the ground was muddy; the gutters were full, and that's why she wanted them cleaned. He begrudgingly got on the ladder to clean the gutters. The ladder slipped in the mud, and he fell, becoming a paraplegic. His wife remained at his bedside and attended to his every need, either through love or guilt. Evan's full-time job was athletic coach in the local high school. His passion was hockey; he knew he could never return to coaching hockey being a paraplegic. Evan wanted to die.

One day Evan went into cardiac arrest and, since I had no order for DNR, I called a Code, and he was successfully resuscitated. He was so upset with the nursing staff on the unit. He would not talk to anybody, especially me. I didn't let him die.

I talked to one of the manufacturers of wheel-chairs and asked if they could put studs on the wheels so Evan could continue coaching hockey. I soon found out that, yes, this was possible. They provided Evan with a free wheel-studded wheel-chair because of his passion for hockey. Once he found out, his whole personality changed. He could see the light at the end of the tunnel, and in this case, that light wasn't going to burnout. He had a future; he could go back to his passion.

I Must Remember to Take July 1ˢᵗ Off

July 1st is when the new residents start. This is an extremely challenging time for any nurse dealing with new doctors who are pretty much clueless. As an ICU nurse, I took excellent care of the ones who introduced themselves, not as Dr. Joe Smith but, "Hi, I'm Joe Smith. I just graduated from medical school (they were referred to as post graduate (PG I) replacing the "intern" status), and now I'm hoping you guys can help me learn as much as I can." I also took care of the first-year residents who weren't as pleasant and insisted they were a lot smarter than the nurses. We all made them come to the unit and write the orders, informing them we couldn't take verbal orders from first-year residents.

One first-year resident, George, was the sweetest kid and very dedicated. He wanted to know as much as he possibly about every patient, what to look for, what were the lab values, and anything we could possibly teach him. He spent many hours bugging me to the point that I sometimes couldn't do my work. He was so tired one day that, sitting at the desk, he fell off the chair and broke it. Some of the nurses and I scooped him up, put him in one of the empty rooms, covered him up, and assured him I would wake him up before the attendings make rounds. Meanwhile I put together some notes about the patients who he usually would be describing on rounds. I covered for him for that night.

I can understand why doctors work long hours as residents so, in the event of an emergency, they can function for long hours because they have done it. However, they all had a learning curve. How much can you learn when you're exhausted, and your brain is not functioning? To me, the practice of long hours in training has always been very questionable. I helped George out; George continued to remember our unit as he progressed through his training and survived.

Spinal cord injury patients were very different than other patients. And sometimes, this was difficult to explain to residents who just rotated for a couple of months through the unit and went on to something else. If they were interested and paid attention, they learned. There were simple differences, such as when the patient had difficulty breathing; we did not raise the head of the bed. We lowered it and placed the patient on his side. Since the muscles of the diaphragm were compromised in spinal cord patients, elevating the head of the bed would make it difficult for them to breathe. Some residents were a little hard to convince since it was common practice to elevate the head of the bed with any respiratory difficulty.

Besides training residents, I also trained new nurses. Betty wanted to be an ICU nurse; a position was available in our spinal cord intensive care unit. Her goal to become one of us. Although she was personable, she was a little slow on the uptake when it came to monitoring the patient. She panicked at the slightest thing. I and some of the other nurses had to calm her down and remind her that you assess the patient, then you go to the machines. Machines were there to help with that assessment but not replace your eyes and ears. With experience, Betty was learning, calming down, and following a routine.

One evening Kathy and I were taking care of our patients in separate rooms when we heard a Code Blue (indicating a cardiac arrest) called for our unit. We both ran out of our rooms to see which patient coded. We found Betty, who was proud of herself because her patient had flatlined on the monitor, and she called the code. I looked at the monitor. The patient had a blood pressure. I rapidly explained to Betty that the patient could not have a blood pressure and a pulse if his heart were not beating. What had happened was one of the ground leads had come off. I reminded her about assessing the patient, not the machine. When the lead was replaced, the patient had a normal cardiac pattern. Meanwhile, we heard the thundering of feet of the Code Team running down the hallway toward our unit. I stuck my head out and yelled, "We got him back. It's OK."

I had a similar experience on my first day on the unit. I had just finished my ICU classes and was eager to try out the equipment. My patient was on a ventilator. I remembered always to check to make sure the lights are all working to identify the problem if an alarm activated. I pushed the button to check the bulbs on the ventilator, and it went blank. My heart sank. I thought the venti-lator had stopped, and the patient was going to die. That didn't happen; one by one, the lights returned, and I realized everything was working fine. I remembered this incident when I advised Betty to check the patient, not the machine.

Joey was one of our problem patients. He would slide his hand under his ventilator tubing connected to his tracheostomy to dislodge the tube. That would cause the alarm to go off. This was his novel way of getting attention instead of using a call light. He had a pressure-sensitive call light that he could activate at any time, however, he felt this would bring the nurses to his bedside a lot faster. This tactic worked because the nurses arrived, thinking there was something wrong with the patient or the ventilator.

I advised Joey many times this is not a good thing to do because if we were busy or didn't hear that alarm, he will remain disconnected and would die. I often wondered if this was Joey's intent. One busy morning at the end of the shift, the residents and attending were making rounds in Joey's room when he disconnected his ventilator tubing again. The residents and attending surgeon were not paying much attention to the ventilator alarm. They ignored the alarm. I noticed, as I was picking up the room with an arm full of laundry that Joey was now in a very slow heart rhythm. The next step would be cardiac arrest. I elbowed my way between the residents and smacked Joey as hard as I could with my fist in his chest. (This technique is called a precordial thump and is used only in emergencies.) I reconnected the ventilator, gave him hundred percent oxygen, and his heart rate came back up. The doctors stood with their mouths hanging open, wondering what just happened. I turned around slowly and said, "He does that a lot" and just moved on. It took me a while to realize what that must have looked like, but it was effective. I later found out Joey was transferred to a long-term facility where he continued his habit of disconnecting his ventilator to get attention. He died there. I believe this was Joey's wish.

Working 12-hour shifts was starting to take its toll on my body. A friend of one of my colleagues was doing home care and asked if I'd be interested in working four days a month to fill in for vacations and just to help. Since I had four days off during the week, I thought I could do this, and it might be interesting to look at a different aspect of nursing. In home care nursing, you are independent in making your calls and spending the time necessary to meet the needs of your patients. It would allow me to do some needed patient teaching and another new opportunity in which to excel, or at least try.

CHAPTER FIFTEEN

HOME CARE NURSING

"Nursing is love in action and there is no finer manifestation of it than the care of the poor and disabled in their own homes."

**— Lillian Wald, founder
Visiting Nurse Service of New York**

SINCE I USUALLY had four days in a row off from my duties in the ICU, I decided to see if home care may be a good fit. Home care nursing had many advantages and disadvantages. It was quite different from the typical nursing environment to which I was accustomed.

After a brief orientation with my supervisor, I went with her on a couple of visits to get the feel of the documentation and to meet a few of her patients. These would be the ones I would be following on her days off, maybe a couple of times a month. I was comfortable with that, and her clients were nice, friendly, and welcoming. The neighborhoods were safe, and their residents were accustomed to visiting nurses.

One of the things to remember is you are in somebody's home, and you respect their environment no matter what it looks like. Some were neat and clean; some looked like they had been ransacked, but again this was their environment, and it was OK.

WHERE IS THE UTILITY ROOM?

One of the apparent issues was that there was no clean or dirty utility room. After all, you are in people's homes, and you must work with what you have available. Sometimes there wasn't a whole lot available, as I soon found out. I carried supplies that I might need in a bag in my car. I was also required to have a section of my trunk designated as a "dirty section" for contaminated items such as blood draws going to the lab. This in part represented clean and dirty utility rooms, except they were in my car. The idea was to separate clean supplies from anything contaminated, just like the hospital. After I thought this through, I was ready to give it a whirl.

One of the tremendous advantages was that I was on my own time. If I wanted to stop to get a cup of coffee between visits, I could do that. If I wanted to get lunch, I could do that. I wasn't held to a scheduled time for a visit as long as I made them unless there was an appointment or a specific time to meet with family. I was on my own.

I soon realized I should chart on the patient's medical record immediately after leaving the patient's home before I forgot all the details. If I wanted to finish my documentation later, I could take it home and do it there. I elected to finish it after each visit.

Most of the supplies I used were simple; I often had an opportunity to suggest materials that were relatively inexpensive and easy for the families or patients to obtain. For instance, I cared for a lady who had incontinence problems. It became costly to use a diaper, a wound cleanser, and harsh material to scrub her bottom every time she had incontinent. A seasoned home care nurse suggested using Barbasol shaving cream from a dollar store. Barbasol was relatively inexpensive and contained a moisturizer that protected the skin from irritation. It had a pleasant odor and worked well as a cleanser.

Another patient had a draining wound that required frequent non-sterile dressing changes. One of the effective methods was to use a cheap sanitary pad, again purchased at a dollar store, which was a lot more cost-effective than using a heavy absorbent dressing. It was about 75% of the cost. This presented a big saving for any family.

Sometimes odor control was an issue; room deodorizers are expensive. Potpourri or even peppermint oil placed on some cotton balls sometimes helped control the odor. Keeping the patient clean and removing material out of the room was the most effective solution.

What Do You Mean You Don't Have It?

I faced a consistent challenge in having the supplies I needed. Some families had a supply of what they would typically use for patient care while others were clueless about what to get or where to get it. Some substitutes were flat out dangerous. Instead of calling for advice, some families got too creative.

For example, a patient had a difficult-to-heal draining wound on her leg. I made a few visits since my background was in wound care. I couldn't understand, with what I was using, why it wasn't healing. When I questioned the patient, she informed me that she was having her dog lick it clean. Her dog looked like it was on death's door, with half of its teeth missing. I can only imagine what bacteria was being deposited in that wound and keeping it from healing. I love my animals, but I certainly wouldn't let them lick my wounds. You have no idea where that tongue has been. Someone years ago told her that her dog's tongue was a good thing, so that's why she did it. This was another opportunity for extensive patient education.

The majority of the patients I visited were glad to see the visiting nurse. Some questioned if a visit was necessary. Some requested me to make stops for them to pick up something on my way to their house. This was against organizational policy. But I did it anyway because I know how difficult it would be for somebody who's homebound with no car and unable to drive to pick up medication. At that time, there were no grocery services that would deliver food supplies. Not everybody has friendly neighbors or relatives.

The patients I saw had a variety of illnesses; some were chronic, some were newly diagnosed, and some were at the end stage of life. For instance, a gentleman had a wife who was diagnosed with terminal cancer and was in hospice care, not expected to live much longer. I spoke with him several times about end of life issues and what to expect when someone is dying. They both knew the diagnosis, were accepting of the future, and just tried to comfort each other as best they could.

When I made my visit one morning, I found his wife sitting on the couch, quite dead. I had mentioned to him that his wife had passed away, and I wasn't sure he noticed. She had no vital signs and was very definitely dead. I asked why he didn't call the phone number that was an emergency number for the visiting nurse. "I knew you were coming in the morning, so I decided to wait. I know she is dead, and she ain't going nowhere." He simply waited for me to show up.

I called the police, who sent a medical examiner to remove the body and do an autopsy to rule out foul play. I also called the home care office; they were surprised the husband had not called. When I called her family physician, he was surprised that he wasn't notified. I informed him that nobody was notified until I arrived. People grieve their losses in different ways. The husband may have wanted to spend his last moments with his wife alone.

My career in home care was short-lived. The most difficult aspect was not having what I needed. There was no central supply. I couldn't run to the closet and pick up something; it was like working with one hand tied behind my back. The seasoned home care nurses I spoke with advised me that they just carried extra things in their car. After a while, I guess you get accustomed to anything.

The patient had a plan of care, the visits are relatively routine, and you couldn't always anticipate what you might need as extra supplies.

Since I was filling in part-time, I wasn't always aware of the plan for every patient. I did what I could and worked with what I had available.While I found the work interesting, it wasn't for me. I liked the convenience of going down the hall and getting what I needed.

I enjoyed the opportunity to do some education with the patients and their families to help them cope with whatever it was they dealing with (that required frequent visits by a visiting nurse). Some were receptive; some were ridiculous with every excuse in the book not to do what was needed.

One visit required me to go into a poor section of Detroit. I had my bag with me when I went to visit an elderly gentleman who lived on the second floor in a two-story small apartment complex. I knocked on his door. He opened the door with a loaded gun aimed at me. He asked, "Hi, who are you?" I told him, "I am the nurse I'm coming here to check your blood pressure." I should have checked mine at the time; I'm sure it rose a little bit! Politely he told me he had a lot of trouble with kids and gangs. I thought, "Oh good, my car is parked out front. I wonder if it'll be there when I finish my visit?"

I checked his blood pressure and went through a little bit of all information on loaded weapons. I told him, "You might get nervous and shoot yourself or somebody could take it away from you and shoot you. If you have problems, you should contact the police." He said, "They all already knew. I don't want to bother anybody. I can take care of my problems." Fortunately, his blood pressure was just fine, but not mine! We parted company, and I wrote a little note in his medical record warning anybody else who followed on this home visit, "Please be careful."

I continued my full-time job in the ICU and still relieved home care nurses during the summer months, on the weekends, a couple of times a month. As the complexity of patients in the ICU increased, the workload and late hours started to take a toll on my body. I decided that intensive care nursing was designed for much younger nurses, and I accepted a position as a manager in a long-term care traumatic brain injury facility. This was another new area of nursing for me to evaluate.

CHAPTER SIXTEEN:

HEALING THE TRAUMATIZED BRAIN WHILE MAKING INSERVICE EDUCATION FUN

"You either get bitter or you get better. It's that simple. You either take what has been dealt to you and allow it to make you a better person, or you allow it to tear you down. The choice does not belong to fate, it belongs to you."

— Josh Shipp

MY EXPERIENCE IN working with traumatic brain injury patients in the ICU led to an opportunity to continue my education in working with traumatic brain injury (TBI) patients going through rehabilitation. I took a job at the Waterford Center, which was known for successes in providing rehabilitation for individuals with traumatic brain injury. The Waterford Center was licensed as a long-term care facility providing rehabilitation mostly to traumatic brain injury patients. It also had a long-term care unit for patients who were sub-acute in a persistent vegetative state, and a unit that was a general nursing long term care environment. I was hired as a manager for the TBI unit.

Years ago, if you were a great nurse, you worked in a hospital. If you were a mediocre skilled nurse, you might work in a doctor's office or clinic. If you were below average, you worked in long term care (in a nursing home).

Over the years, that has changed drastically. Today's long term care patients are in various stages of needing acute nursing care such as ventilators or complex intravenous feedings. The patients at Waterford were of the sub-acute rehabilitation variety. They had brain injury and needed to work with therapies – physical, recreational, occupational, speech, neuropsychiatry, and vocational rehabilitation – to get them back to as much of a mental functioning level as possible. There were several RNs on staff, several LPNs, and an incredible group of nursing assistants who amazed me with their ability to get these somewhat uncooperative patients dressed, undressed, toileted, bathed, and fed. They were indeed something to behold.

UNDERSTANDING THE BEHAVIOR

Traumatic brain injury patients are generally classified by their behavior and level of understanding. In 1974, a group of speech pathologists at Rancho Los Amigos Hospital in California decided to group these categories into classifications rather than repeating their observations every time they documented. That became the Rancho Los Amigos Scale for traumatic brain injury, and it's as follows:

- Level I: no response, in a comatose state

- Level II: generalized response

- Level III: localized response

- Level IV: confused-agitated

- Level V: confused and inappropriate

- Level VI: confused and appropriate

- Level VII: automatic and appropriate

- Level VIII: purposeful and appropriate

Once the staff understood and categorized these behaviors, we could anticipate the patients' needs and conduct. Their behaviors weren't always safe, like psychiatric patients with poor judgment.

Knowing the unpredictability of the patient allowed the nurse to anticipate where a problem may occur.

Patients learned there are consequences to their actions. For example, before admission, Jason tried to jump onto an elevator that was between floors, slipped, and fell down the elevator shaft about 10 stories. Hitting his head, Jason was in a coma for almost two years and came to us for rehabilitation. It was amazing to watch the occupational therapist work with him to be able to bring him around with stimulation, such as a feather on his face to see if he would reach for it. Certain scents like cherry placed on his lips elicited a licking or sucking response.

Eventually, Jason reached the Rancho Level IV, and that was the behavior problem level. Jason was powerful. He ripped the wallpaper off the walls in his room. That was OK; I hated it anyway, and it didn't do much to calm patients since it was covered with huge clusters of roses. He took the binding off his mattress, all the way around, ripping the heavy plastic with his bare hands. If Jason liked you, he tried to hug you but because he was extremely strong, he could break your ribs.

Jason had a Tickle Me Elmo toy, which was his buddy. When Jason misbehaved, we took Tickle

Me Elmo away for a short period. When he recognized he did something wrong, we would give Elmo back to him.

Jason progressed to the point that he could feed himself. He remained a serious behavioral issue and was eventually discharged to a behavioral group home dealing with traumatic brain injury patients.

I learned a lot about the basics of what was important to Jason and other patients with TBI. These patients required help with their basic needs for food, shelter, and warmth. When this was done, they gradually progressed to needing human contact, conversation, and stimuli but not overstimulation. It was amazing to see the progress patients made in a seemingly short time with extensive rehabilitation.

We had another individual who was in a severe car accident. Juan was the unbelted driver of the car. He exited the car through the rear window, headfirst, so you can imagine the force of impact. He was somewhere around a Rancho level VI. Although Juan understood he had head and neck injuries, he didn't know where he was or why he was at Waterford. He kept asking for a suit because he had to go to a meeting; he was challenging to re redirect.

After several months of work, we could see Juan was almost normal in his thinking and behavior. This was to the credit of the folks working with rehab and recreational therapy, getting him to socialize at an appropriate level. This was truly amazing work.

Another interesting patient, Pierre had a flashback to his military service and decided to guard the only elevator against anybody coming on or getting off. He was ready with his "bayonet" ballpoint pen. He tried to stab anyone who dared to enter his guard post. The assistant administrator, Mr. Bellows, was a large man 6 foot 2, around 250 pounds with snow-white hair. The only way we could get Pierre to leave his post and be reassigned to his bed was to have his "commanding officer" (AKA Mr. Bellows) give him a direct order. When Mr. Bellows approached him and said, "Stand at attention, soldier", Pierre snapped to attention while saluting Mr. Bellows. Mr. Bellows immediately ordered our patient back to his bed for rest and to await further orders. Pierre immediately saluted, turned around, and headed for his room after relinquishing his "bayonet". Thank goodness for big and military-looking individuals! I wondered what would have happened if the plan with Mr. Bellows didn't work as expected. Who then would come to our rescue?

HEALING THE WOUNDS

The patients who had an injury serious enough to damage their brains usually had wounds some place. Either they were caused by immobility creating pressure injuries on various parts of the anatomy, or cuts, scrapes, abrasions that occurred at the time of the original trauma. I had a lot of patients with wounds. Wound care was one of my specialties; I was quite successful in healing a lot of severe wounds.

One memorable patient had her entire abdominal skin affected by necrotizing fasciitis. It looked as if someone had taken a knife and peeled off her skin. It healed to the extent that when we sent her out for a skin graft, the hospital sent her back, stating she didn't need it.

 Another unfortunate lady got her car pinned between a utility pole and another car during a high-speed police chase. Jaycee sustained significant deep tissue injury to her entire back. Her injury progressed to open wounds in various areas, particularly her buttocks. We treated Jaycee's wounds daily, but they showed little progress due to her deep tissue injury.

Jaycee was beginning to develop a temperature and early signs of sepsis. Her wounds needed immediate debridement (surgical removal of dead tissue). Our case manager, Julie, was able to make arrangements for transfer to the hospital for immediate surgical intervention. I received a message from the hospital that the debridement was successful, and had we waited one more day, Jaycee might have been dead from sepsis. That was a real eye-opener. The staff credited me with saving her life.

Sam Jaffee, the owner of Waterford Center, noticed my skill in wound healing. I had a small office, which was a converted patient's room on the first floor. One day Sam came in, took his sock and shoe off, and placed his foot on my desk, and asked, "Does this look like a problem?" I looked at him and remarked that I was glad he did not have hemorrhoids. What he had was the start of an ingrown toenail, which was easy to fix.

Sam was a bit of a character. He knew the patients and their families, and he had no hesitancy solving disputes if patients were uncooperative with treatment and families interfered. It was a tough job, but somebody had to do it.

For instance, a lady had continuous complaints about her daughter's care. Her daughter's care was appropriate, and her needs were met. I think part of the problem was mom didn't understand what those needs were and how they were to be met. I did the best I could but was unable to please her no matter what I did.

Sam called a meeting to discuss some of these concerns. The concerns were frivolous. It was almost impossible to meet her demands. He suggested that she take her daughter elsewhere. The lady became quite belligerent and said, "How dare you throw my daughter out!" Sam very calmly looked at her, and he said, "Yes, I can, I own the facility, and if you're not happy here, be happy elsewhere." The lady didn't think that was possible. She insisted that she was staying until she was good and ready, and that did not happen. The daughter was ultimately transferred to another facility; I hoped their care was as good as ours.

It was evident that a lot of education needed to occur to have a good understanding of traumatic brain injury and the ramifications for such individuals. That appeared to be my next job.

Take 2 ...and Action

I applied for and received a grant to do a set of videos on the different levels of traumatic brain injury. They were to serve as a guide for nurses who are not familiar with TBI, patients, and for the family so they understand the patient's behavior. Families were often embarrassed by some patients' lack of inhibition. The first thing you would hear them say was, "They never acted like that before." Watching the video allowed families to understand how the brain heals and how long it would take. That was a tremendous help.

Our local public television station had a series on the brain. I approached them with my project and asked if I could use some of the segments. They were gracious and told me, "Sure, use whatever you want." I was surprised and grateful.

Waterford hired a company that came in and did the filming. Originally they wanted a script and actors to portray our patients, and I insisted we use our own staff who had a much better appreciation and knowledge of the behavior of traumatic brain-injured individuals. The company was impressed with my directing and producing abilities. I had a ball. We laughed so hard because of course, my staff did ham it up a bit, but we got the point across, and the videos were a tremendous help. I also applied for continuing education units (CEU) for the nurses who reviewed the videos, and 3.5 CEUs were granted. I received highly positive feedback from everybody who watched the videos. It was an interesting and rewarding project.

One person who benefited was the wife of the delightful little gentleman who was a deacon in his church. Because of his level of brain injury, he was left with no inhibitions and did whatever he felt like doing no matter what or where. He was confused, and he had a nasty problem of swearing like a sailor. His wife was mortified. The pastor and people from the church wanted to come to visit, and she said, "They can't, they just can't." Once we explained to her and had her watched the videos, she had a better understanding of why her husband was acting the way he was.

I wore many hats at the Waterford Center, including wound care specialist, clinical nurse consultant, education specialist, and an interim Director of Nursing. I built on my experience but did not find being Director of Nursing engaging. I turned down the position when our former director left, but I did help until they found a replacement and that, thank God, didn't take long.

HOW TO GET THEM TO SHARE MY PASSION AND OTHER MYTHS OF NURSING INSERVICE EDUCATION

I was always involved in some type of staff education. I believed education was necessary; if they understood why they were doing something, they would do a better job. That often proved to be accurate and became my mantra throughout my nursing career. When it came to staff education at Waterford it was challenging to make it enjoyable. I wanted them to share my passion. Their interest, however, was not in sharing my passion but often getting out of an educational session and returning to patient care. I understand that, I know tasks must be completed; patients' call lights must be answered, and people need what they need. I wanted to educate them so they could work smarter rather than harder. Unfortunately, my enthusiasm wasn't always shared by everybody.

On the units, I frequently grabbed nurses to educate them on wound care as the opportunity presented itself. I thought that was usually well accepted. Many years later, I ran into a nurse while shopping. She said, "When the nurses saw you coming down the hall they would hide for fear of more education." Oh well, at least I tried.

Even Doctors Need A Current BLS Card

It was a requirement that anyone in health care throughout all hospitals and facilities was required to have a current Basic Life Support (BLS) training, renewable every 2 years. The education was in place, based on research, to provide emergent care in the case of heart attack, whether it was a patient or possibly a staff member, visitor, or anyone else. I was a certified instructor with the American Heart Association and taught the class periodically for the staff and in the community.

Our medical staff also were required to have a current BLS card. Our staff educator refused to teach them; she was very intimidated by the doctors. I was old enough that nothing intimidated me, including doctors. They were interested in learning the latest American Heart Association guidelines and were just as nervous passing their test as any student on the planet taking a test. Being a doctor didn't always help. Their resuscitative techniques were quite good, and they passed with flying colors. This was to my great relief, as I was the teacher.

I must have done an excellent job because the following day, I heard from our medical director, Dr. Howard Canal, on his life-saving effort in his office. An elderly female patient was in the exam room, waiting to be seen. When he walked in the room, the poor lady was asleep and was just leaning her head back against the wall with her mouth open. He yelled out to the staff to call 911 and shook her yelling, "Annie, Annie are you OK?" (Annie was the name of our practice resuscitation manikin). She looked at him and said, "My name is not Annie, it's Sarah." I guess he got the message. He immediately canceled the 911 call.

One of the other physicians said he was at dinner with his wife, and he noticed another diner was choking. He calmly got up, went over to the table, and performed the Heimlich maneuver, popping out a piece of meat. Then he came back and finished his dinner with his wife. She was amazed. I guess the education wasn't a waste of time.

FEED THEM AND THEY WILL COME

Never underestimate the power of donuts. I discovered when I brought food, my attendance was increased for my inservice classes regardless of the topic. Our nurse educator Marcy moved on to another position, and I took over her role. Sitting through lectures can be boring, so, with my warped sense of humor, I managed to keep their attention and get people interested in what's going on. The staff was not always enthusiastic about participating in education that required a hands-on demonstration. I tried to incorporate as many senses into my presentations to grab and keep their attention. What worked best was the stories and the jokes I shared. If nothing else, they came for the entertainment and, in the process, learned something.

The Waterford Center also had five group homes. Each home was dedicated to long-term care of brain-injured patients with a variety of needs. Some homes had patients working part-time, leaving the facility, and returning in the evening. Other homes catered to individuals in a persistent vegetative state. When able, residents received vocational training to obtain jobs such as assembling some parts, stocking grocery shelves, stuffing envelopes, and doing other jobs according to their ability to participate and be successful. This provided an income as well.

There were rules in the group homes that had to be followed. Everyone had a job. They had a private room that needed to be maintained clean and orderly. The medication was dispensed by the staff, so I periodically had classes for them on medication administration, the typical side effects, and what potential side effects needed to be monitored.

Every year, our medical director made rounds and did a physical exam on all the group home residents. I often met him at the group home to assist where I could. During a visit on a cold winter day, I ran out to the car to get an article I wanted to share with Dr. Canal. I did not take my coat. The car was parked right outside the building. Unfortunately, I slipped on some ice and fell and couldn't get up. I was lying next to my car, wondering if this would be how my life would end, frozen to death in the middle of a snowbank. I did not have a cell phone with me; it didn't do any good to yell because I was a distance from the door. Eventually, somebody noticed that I wasn't there, so they went outside and there I was lying in a very cold heap of snow. A few people ran out help me up and got me inside to warm me up. Another important lesson learned; don't go outside in cold weather without a coat even if it's a short distance.

As our census dropped, my life at Waterford was coming to an end. The position closed because I was expensive. I did such a good job on training everybody; Sam felt he could probably do without me. I understood it was not personal, just business.

I was offered a full-time position as a nurse educator with the St. Basil Health System. The hospital was relatively close to home, and I was very tempted, but I didn't want to take a chance of having another job disappear on me. It's happened too many times. I wanted to get into something a lot more stable. One of my college professors once told me that there's two ways to lose your job: one was to be very bad at it, and the other was to be very good at it. I must've fallen in the very good part. During that time and for many years, I was a clinical nursing instructor for County Community College in their nursing program.

I decided to finish my master's in nursing and teach nursing full time. Since a master's in nursing was required, I went back to school. I already had a master's degree in healthcare administration and found many of my credits were transferrable. The University asked me to teach some classes in the administration division. I taught a few classes, and that assisted me with my tuition. I doubled and tripled my class load to finish as soon as possible. I graduated with a 4.0 average and continued to teach part-time for the University in management. The national nursing honor society Sigma Theta Tau International invited me to join. I was quite honored.

I continued to teach part-time at the University in nursing and management. I soon learned that a full-time faculty position was available at County Community College. I was familiar with their nursing program since I had been teaching clinical students for several years. I interviewed and accepted a full-time faculty position. I love to talk. So, teaching in front of a classroom was in no way intimidating. I was eager to share my experiences and, at the very least, had a captive audience for my stories. I was eager to move on to my next venture in nursing.

CHAPTER SEVENTEEN:

CHALLENGES OF ACADEMIA

"The harder you work for something, the greater you feel when you achieve it."

— Susan Johanson, RN

COUNTY COMMUNITY COLLEGE offered educational opportunities to thousands of students. The nursing program began in the 1970s and took place on two campuses. I was familiar with the Nursing Department since I had been teaching clinical nursing since 1993. The Dean notified me there was an open full-time faculty position, and asked if I would be interested. Yes, I definitely would be interested since, at the time, I was unemployed except for teaching at the University. I was quite excited!

I have a passion for sharing my experiences and knowledge, and let's face it, molding those mushy minds into good nurses was a great ego trip. Finally, I would be teaching a captive audience; like it or not, they would have to listen to what I had to say.

Nursing education is quite different in today's world from what it was when I was a student nurse. I couldn't teach the same way I learned: the instructor talked, and everybody took notes, and the faster they spoke, the faster you wrote. Heaven forbid your pencil should break.

I much preferred to lecture using stories, pictures, and examples of the topic I was teaching about rather than just expecting students to jot down words and memorize them. If they didn't understand the concept, they would never remember it no matter how hard they tried. My son Ryan, the IT guru, was instrumental in assisting me with the development of colorful PowerPoint slides to demonstrate the subject. I was also able to incorporate some videos to enforce the visual impact.

I was new to full-time teaching and soon learned that the politics in health care paled compared to the politics in academia. There were so many deans and associate deans, some with overlapping responsibilities and unclear reporting structure. Although it seemed like I had been in school all my life, it's different being on the other end, being the instructor.

I remember walking into my first class and seeing all those wide-eyed students. Wow! This was a different feeling seeing all those eager faces staring at me, waiting for me to impart knowledge. I loved to be entertaining, so lecturing was no problem. I was prepared for the subject matter since I worked the majority of my life in orthopedics or with brain-injured patients, both in acute trauma and sub-acute long term care, and those were the two major areas about which I taught.

That wasn't, however, where I started. I taught a fundamentals of nursing class. It had been a long, long time since I took my own fundamentals class, and it was obvious to me this was going to be more demanding than I had thought. Some students possessed good manual dexterity and could draw up medication in a syringe with no difficulty. Wrapping a blood pressure cuff around an arm and taking the blood pressure took a lot more practice. Others were totally all thumbs, but they wanted to be a nurse. They had the desire, and I had the stamina to make that happen.

There wasn't an orientation for new faculty members, so I winged it. I had enough academia in my life to know how to write a decent exam.

When I created my first test, I put together a "fill in the blanks" quiz, not rocket science, that could have two or three correct but different responses. I wanted to evaluate the students' thought processes, how they arrived at their response. Inadvertently I passed out the answer key. When I got it back, I was looking at this one student's writing next to what looked like mine. It was mine! He had proceeded to correct the answer key. I explained to him that these were the correct answers. He included his rationale for why he thought the answers were incorrect and why he responded as he did. While his rationale was interesting, it had utterly no scientific background. At least he was thinking. His former occupation was a UPS driver. There were a lot of nurses in his family who were pushing him towards a nursing career. His heart wasn't in it; it just wasn't his calling. He returned to his previous job.

Student Nurses Are Fun to Watch Most of the Time

I advanced from the trials and tribulations of the Fundamentals course. I wanted to teach students based on my knowledge of the specialty areas. While the newbies were interesting, I didn't have the patience. Next, I progressed to the first medical-surgical class, with patient assignments and a perioperative experience. That meant taking the students into the operating room so they could observe sterile technique, teamwork in the OR, and some of the common surgeries. It was important for the students to observe the procedures to better understand why their patient was in so much pain post-op.

In the operating room, you never know what students are going to do. I instructed them, "Do not touch anything. Do not bug anybody. You are there to observe. Stand up against the wall where you will have a good view of the procedure." Most of the nurses were happy to see students and were glad to share their experiences. The staff informed them on what was taking place during the operation. Most of the doctors were welcoming to students, after all, they were students at some point, and for some, that was a recent experience.

One of my students was fascinated with a Bair Hugger (a forced-air warming blanket). This is a thin plastic blanket that fills up with air and warms the patient. She went over and put her ungloved hands on it, saying, "Wow, this is really soft and warm." Because this was sterile equipment, no one was happy she touched it with her hands. All the sterile drapes were torn down, and everything was re-draped, causing a delay in surgery. My student must have missed that part about "do not touch anything".

As time went on, it was challenging to find appropriate surgical observation opportunities for the students. I resorted to the Internet. I found several websites that showed a variety of surgical procedures the students could observe in the classroom. This was a big help and a lot less dangerous than having students delay surgery or distract the surgeon. Some websites had a surgeon describe step-by-step what was going on during the operation.

I continued lecturing and observing the students in clinical areas. While for some, it was difficult to grasp the concepts, some excelled because they studied and had a better foundation. I often said learning nursing was like learning to drive a car. It was all new. The first day you got behind the wheel of the car, you had to judge if you should put your foot on the brake or keep going when you approached a light. Now you drive yourself to school eating a taco; and you arrive in one piece. Nursing function eventually becomes somewhat automatic once the students learn their skills and build on a solid foundation. I encouraged the students to identify their passion, work in that discipline, and be happy.

 I rotated to several different hospitals so students would get the best experience possible. My next assignment was to teach cardiology, respiratory diseases, and hematology, substituting for an instructor who was on medical leave. The instructor shared her lecture notes but not her exams. So again, with the help of my son Ryan, I was able to put together some creative questions to test the students' retention of my lectures. The students were surprised by my approach.

After the first exam, one of the students approached the Dean with a complaint about me. The Dean was rather surprised since she knew me quite well for many years. Her complaint was rather simple: "I paid five hundred dollars for the other teacher's exam, and Mrs. Conklin didn't use it. How dare she? That cost me a lot of money!" The Dean could not believe her ears. She suggested the student ask for a refund. I'm not sure the student was smart enough to be a nurse. There were ramifications for the student's deceptive activities. She was given a second chance, passed her exams, and managed to graduate. There's no wiggle room for cheating when lives depend on the nurse's knowledge.

I had a clear understanding of the anatomy of the heart and dysfunctions due to my experiences with open heart surgery at the Cleveland Clinic. Reading an EKG and teaching life-threatening arrhythmias to students was a little more demanding. We covered the pathophysiology of heart disease, pulmonary disease, and related laboratory findings. They were motivated to learn, and I was excited to teach.

I would often look at my class during lectures and visualize light bulbs above each student's head: some were 40W, some were 60W, some were burned out, and some had triple levels. It was fascinating to keep them inspired. Occasionally a nonfunctioning lightbulb lit up when the student had a question. At least they were awake. I covered a lot of information in that class. Some students did exceptionally well, while others struggled. Each student had a mentor to assist with study skills, test-taking skills, and occasionally dealing with personal matters interfering with pursuing their education.

The Dean approached me in October to cover for a clinical rotation due to a sudden illness of the instructor. Unfortunately, this was a day rotation, and I was unable to cover a day rotation due to my full-time job. I could include an afternoon rotation if the change could be made. The school was quick to accommodate me and notified all the students that they must report to the lobby of the hospital at 4 PM since their clinical rotation had changed.

I arrived early, sat in the lobby, waited for my students, and started to read the newspaper. Occasionally I would look up to see if everyone had shown up. To my surprise, I heard one of my disgruntled students complaining, "Who does she think she is? I have plans for Halloween, and now I can't do anything. I have to be in clinical!"

Some of the students joined the pity party, and I occasionally lowered my paper to see if everybody had arrived. When I counted my allotted number of students, I put down the paper and introduced myself as their instructor. Oops, I saw a lot of jaws drop. This is going to be a fun semester, I could tell. The students looked a bit horrified, and they should have been. It was an important lesson for the students — watch what you say because you never know who's listening. Clinical rotation proceeded as expected. The students worked hard to overcome their first-day experiences meeting their instructor.

In the clinical areas, I always asked the staff nurses to let me know if there were a procedure on the unit or anything the students would benefit from by observing. These students had some experience with clinical nursing, having completed one medical-surgical class, and some had an obstetric (OB) rotation at that point. Their knowledge, however, wasn't always evident. For example, a patient needed a Foley catheter changed. The students should be able to do this with little difficulty. I asked who was willing to do the procedure, and they knew if they didn't volunteer I would volunteer them.

One of the students said she would be more than happy to do it. Our patient was a 90-year-old female who had been in the hospital for some time. When we approached the bed, we noticed her respirations were rather odd, almost like Cheyne-Stokes respirations (an abnormal pattern of breathing, characterized by deeper and sometimes faster breathing followed by no breath). I asked the staff nurse caring for this patient if there was a "do not resuscitate order" due to her age. The nurse stated the patient was a full code, meaning she needed to be resuscitated if her heart stopped. I strongly suggested she call a Code since a cardiac arrest appeared to be eminent. Even my students recognized that this patient was dying. I sent my students to get the crash cart and clear out unnecessary furniture in the room. The nurse returned and stated the patient was okay and proceeded to show me a monitor strip indicating that the patient was in ventricular fibrillation, a life-threatening arrhythmia. The patient was not okay! This nurse did not recognize the arrhythmia. I went to the nurses' station and called the Code. As the team approached, one of my students, a paramedic, was ready to go ahead and intubate the patient. I had to remind her that it was not her role at this point, and the anesthesiologist would take over. The patient was resuscitated and survived. However, the catheter change was delayed for obvious reasons.

But it was an essential lesson for the students; if you don't know what you are doing, go find somebody who does because you should never put yourself in a situation where you're the only one with brains. Network early in your career and continue throughout your career. If you're working in a cardiac unit, find out who's good at reading EKG's. You will find your niche as you go on in life. As a nurse, you develop a 6th sense that tells you when you're about to get into trouble and also keeps you out of trouble. Unless you know where to get help, you can rather rapidly find yourself in a disastrous situation. It was a good lesson for them and for everybody, including the staff nurse, who, by the way, was an agency nurse and not familiar with cardiac patients. It wasn't apparent why she was assigned to a monitored floor if she couldn't interpret a rhythm on the monitor.

My student Leroy took my instructions quite literally. He was a former engineer who lost his job and decided to go into nursing so he could help people. He was very dedicated but thought like an engineer, one thing at a time. His patient returned from a procedure, and he knew that he had to get the vital signs, a typical routine aspect of care post-procedure. This patient was rather boisterous and demanded his pain medication, which the staff nurse said she would get to him as soon as she could. That wasn't good enough. He contacted his homies, who brought him some street drugs. Right on their heels were the police trying to do a drug bust. As they were wrestling to get the drugs and the individual who brought them in custody, my student elbowed his way to the patient to get his blood pressure. I tried to tell him in a nice way, "You know things are a little busy right now at the bedside; it can wait a while". Everybody was screaming. I pointed out that the patient's blood pressure might be a little elevated, and you might want to wait a few minutes until things settle down. It became one of those teachable moments.

Another one of my earlier students, Crystal, had a Hospice patient. It was an opportunity for the whole clinical group to experience the end of life and talk more about what to expect in the dying process. The patient was actively dying; the husband was there and knew death was imminent. It wasn't a surprise for anyone. The family was relieved knowing her suffering would soon end.

I was on the phone with pharmacy checking on an order when the student came to me, pulling my sleeve, and calling my name. I finished with the pharmacy and asked her, "What is your problem that couldn't wait?" She blurted out, "My patient is dead!" I asked her, "What makes you think your patient is dead?" She responded, "She's not breathing; she has no pulse, and she looked dead." I accompanied her back to the patient's bedside, and we discussed the next steps. We comforted the husband and started gathering the patient's belongings. The student was in tears, and I felt sorry for her, as this was her first experience with a dying patient. I suggested we notify the doctor, and we would discuss death and dying in post clinical conference. She was somewhat relieved when the husband thanked her for taking care of his wife and the fact that his wife was no longer in pain.

I eventually found my niche and taught about bones and brains: orthopedics, neurological diseases, and continuum of care, including long term care and rehabilitation. My students were ready to graduate. Some were excited to finally see the light at the end of the tunnel, while others were rather burned out. They couldn't wait to get out, find a job, and start making money. They lost some of their enthusiasm for learning.

Sharing the Knowledge without Scaring Them

Since these students were about to graduate, I would incorporate a lot of their previous knowledge into case studies and into what I was teaching. I focused on the basics of nursing care: "You cannot replace your eyeballs, ears, or five senses when it comes to observation. What do you smell when you walk into the room? Is there a foul odor? From where is it coming? Investigate it!" I talked about some of the disasters, both natural and unnatural, that may affect the patient. I advised them it was essential, no matter where they worked, to know the emergency protocols. I shared some of my hair-raising experiences. I asked them, "You're not going to look for the emergency manual when you have a fire, so, where are your fire pull stations? Does your unit have oxygen piped into the walls, and are there instructions how to shut it off in case of a fire? Is your life-saving equipment (like a ventilator) plugged into an outlet plug where, if you lost power, a generator would still supply energy? These are things that you don't think of until you're faced with it. It can and will be terrifying! You always need to plan ahead. It wasn't raining when Noah built the ark."

I taught the students to incorporate critical thinking in their patient assessment. Critical thinking is taught in every aspect of nursing regardless of what school they attended and at every level of nursing education. For some students, it's a hard concept to understand. It's really quite simple. I explained the easiest way to understand this concept is to look at your patient. As a nurse, you already know the patient's diagnosis, and you could anticipate what problems may be related to that illness. Based on that diagnosis and your assessment, you consider what potential problems or complications may arise while under your care. You then proceed to formulate a plan to avoid the situations from happening. It may be as simple as monitoring your patient more closely or moving the crash cart closer to your patient's room in case you need it. Anticipating any disaster and having the necessary equipment at hand is the best thing to keep a critical situation from becoming a disaster.

It was challenging to teach students how to prioritize. Where do you start? That's something I covered in lecture and particularly in the clinical areas. I assigned most students one patient, then two or three depending on their ability to prioritize and manage time. Since this was their last medical-surgical clinical rotation, they needed to be ready for the real world. One of the things I emphasized to everybody was that time management and organization take time to develop. No one can organize you. If you see an organized nurse, observe her method of getting ready for the shift. How does she prioritize? The need to create priorities is often a problem encountered by new graduates and an impatient preceptor. I warned the students they might have to remind their preceptor that everybody had their first day in any career or job and with the proper guidance survived and improved.

Prioritization wasn't that difficult to teach. I had one noteworthy student, Rosie, who was extremely disorganized. She knew her patient needed assistance with meals. Once the tray arrived in the room, Rosie opened the lid and saw that the food was cold. She walked to the pantry to warm the meal. When she returned with the meal, she forgot to take the soup, which was also cold. That led to another trip to the pantry with the soup. Upon returning with the soup, which was now hot, Rosie had to assist the patient in getting into a position to eat the hot soup. Once she helped the patient with a bowl of hot soup, Rosie again went to warm the meal. And then there was the coffee, also lukewarm – another trip to the pantry.

When I observed her many trips, I finally asked her, "What are you doing?" She informed me she was trying to get her patient through the meal. At the rate she was going, dinner would be completed somewhere around breakfast time. I suggested she look at the items on the tray, decide what needed to be warm, and take everything at one time to warm it. Rosie eventually picked up speed, but I was concerned about other areas where she demonstrated a lack of critical thinking.

Rosie and I had a chat. She informed me she was on medication for mental health issues, but another instructor told her to stop taking her meds because they might make her sleepy. This advice was not a good idea without her doctor's approval. I wasn't worried about Rosie being sleepy; I was worried about Rosie not thinking in a critical situation. She resumed her medications, and by the time her clinical rotation was complete, Rosie demonstrated a safe level of competence.

As part of the clinical rotation, I assigned the students to do a teaching plan to clarify either the diagnosis, medications the patient would be discharged with, or any information the patient needed about the disease process, complications, and so on. Carlos was an enthusiastic student dedicated to patient teaching. A student after my own heart! He also felt that education was essential to keep the patient from developing complications. I agreed.

When Carlos created a teaching plan for a newly diagnosed diabetic, his plan was based on the diagnosis and the details the patient needed to know. His extensive plan covered how diabetes affects the body, signs and symptoms of high and low blood sugar, medications, diet, and the importance of exercise and of keeping track of blood sugars. His plan covered everything you've ever wanted to know about diabetes. Unfortunately, any patient would be overwhelmed trying to understand it.

I suggested Carlos start by asking the patient, "What you want to know about diabetes?" Start from there. Then proceed to what your patient needs to know, what is nice to know, and leave out what is nuts to know! When you answer the patient's immediate burning questions, he'll tend to listen to whatever else you have to say. Carlos narrowed his plan considerably and was able to supply his patient with resources and literature to review at his own pace. He did an excellent job; the patient was grateful.

SCARING THEM, IT'S OKAY

I had a simple criterion for judging the competence of my students. If I'm in a hospital, ready to slip into a coma, and see you as my nurse, do I close my eyes and slip into that coma because I know you will take care of me, or do I gather my last ounce of strength and get out of there? They seem to understand that concept. Some instructors felt you must be strict and judgmental about the skills of the students in the clinical area. This demeanor, they argued, was critical for their development as practitioners.

I had a different philosophy. I believed that if you are approachable, your student will come to you with questions. If you are unapproachable, and they fear to go to you, then they will do what they think is right. It might *not* be. I didn't coddle the students. I gave them honest answers and believed it was okay for the instructor not to know everything, but, as an instructor, you should know where to find the answer.

Teaching in the Google age is another challenge. I asked a question in class, and everybody Googled the answer! I reminded everybody that there's no Google at the bedside. If you understand, you will never forget it. If you memorize it for the sake of just getting through the class or getting through the exam, you will have a problem recalling what to do next.

When I lectured, I liked to tell stories. It is a method of education called *narrative pedagogy*. Later some of my former students told me they didn't always remember what I said to do, but they remembered the stories of what somebody did or what happened, and they followed that. At least the information got to them, and somewhere along the line, they acted appropriately.

I had them share their stories, and their questions from their clinical experiences since the class was divided into multiple hospitals and different clinical instructors. Unless knowledge is applied, it is useless. Not being able to use it safely and appropriately is also meaningless.

I'm a firm believer that all students come to the fountain of knowledge. Some drink; some just gargle. My job was to keep them thirsty. The more examples I could incorporate into the subject material I covered, the easier it was for them to understand. When I spoke about using assistive devices in orthopedic such as walkers, crutches, and canes, I demonstrated that. I had to keep them thirsty somehow.

Chairing a Faculty Meeting Is Like Herding Cats

Soon after I became a full-time faculty member, the faculty voted to elect me as the head of the curriculum committee. It was an opportunity to work on the curriculum and make sure it was current, review any changes step by step, and show the progress from one class to the other from the beginning to graduation. That sounded like an easy task. We met on the third Wednesday of the month from 9 AM to 11 AM. I submitted the agenda in advance, so everybody knew the plans for the meeting, and, most of the time, I personally took the minutes to make sure they were accurate. That task was soon relieved by a dedicated secretary. I was glad for the help.

Trying to get everybody to show up at the meeting on time and contribute according to the agenda, rather than their own agendas, became a challenge. We used Roberts Rules of Order. It soon became evident that a lot of instructors didn't know what that was.

At one point, I tried to put together an agenda with time limits assigned to the topics. If someone wanted to speak longer on any subject, they would have to borrow minutes from a different topic to keep us on track to finish on time. That worked for a while, but not long. It seemed that everybody came to the meeting with their own agendas regardless of what issues were on the agenda. That was an ordeal for 10 years, and, after some health issues, I turned it over to a colleague. Although I was not very successful in changing people, somehow, someway, we all survived. Another lesson learned: work with what you've got. It's not always going to be what you want. I don't want you to misunderstand. I had a dedicated faculty; some were just more dedicated than others. That's the same in any business, job, or career.

Our student population was interesting as well. The enrollment represented numerous countries in our classrooms such as Canada, Romania, Gambia, Western Africa, Japan, Korea, Russia, Poland, Mexico, and New Guinea. All these cultures had their health practices as well as their healthcare beliefs. It was interesting to hear from the students what those cultural practices were regarding health and disease.

I had two students who were brothers, Atta and Bento. Atta graduated and went on for his master's degree, and his younger brother, Bento, was in my class. Their goal was to go back to Gambia where they were planning to start a school of nursing. I gave Atta a lot of my older nursing texts and whatever I could scrounge up to help them put together their dreams. Atta and his brother went back to Gambia. However, I have not heard from them, so I hope they are doing well.

WE ALL HAVE ISSUES

Many of our students were single parents juggling family, transportation, and study times. It was challenging to have all three in order, so most of them needed a Plan B. When life started to interrupt their grades, we put them in the mentoring program. The mentor assisted them in finding out where the issues were and how we, as a faculty, can help them achieve success in our nursing program. The nursing department started an "Early and Often Program" that identified students who were struggling with failing grades, attendance problems, transportation problems, and so on. The program alerted the student's mentor and the administration that the student needed help. The students met with their mentors to further identify what the issues were keeping them from success.

Students did not always know about the available college resources. We made every effort to assist the students in successfully graduating. Outside organizations often provided financial help. The college supplied a variety of programs for those struggling with test-taking skills, organization, and time management.

Nursing was a second or even third career for a lot of our students. Their ages ranged anywhere from 18 years old to my oldest student, who was 56. We had several generations represented with a lot of experience or lack thereof. They all had issues of one sort or another. The expectations were clear:

1. Arrive at clinical on time and do not miss any clinical schedule assignments.
2. Turn in homework when it is due.
3. Be prepared to take the test at the required date and time.

The students could create many excuses for doing absolutely nothing on time. Excuses were not acceptable, and after all, they needed discipline and reliability to function effectively in a health-care setting. When it came to time management, I stressed punctuality as it was an essential factor in the real world when they finally gained employment as a nurse.

I went over the results of the exam, explaining answers. I allowed students to ask questions regarding the validity of the exam questions or to challenge why I marked their answers as wrong. Some of their rationale and concepts were fascinating to listen to, however wrong. I needed to clarify their thinking before they went on their way with their versions of the proper protocols.

BACK TO THE UNIVERSITY

A friend of mine approached me to teach a class at St. Adrian University on legal aspects of healthcare administration and the regulatory process. That sounded like fun. I had some time since I was at the campus only three days a week with my teaching responsibilities, not including the hours I spent at home in preparation. I was always fascinated with how the rules and regulations came about in the legal process in general. I had my master's in administration and was more than willing to share my knowledge and my experiences.

I didn't have an extensive legal background, so I decided to join a chapter of the American Association of Legal Nurse Consultants to obtain knowledge of how the legal system impacts healthcare management. When I was ready, I took an exam to become certified as a legal nurse consultant. The certification exam covered all aspects of the legal process and how it pertained to nurses, and the input nurses can provide during a litigation process. It was quite interesting. There was a lot of information that I could share teaching this class. Certification added to my credibility and qualifications to at least identify potential pitfalls for managers and staff in a healthcare environment.

The students were great; I enjoyed teaching the class in a classroom environment, which I much preferred. I wanted to see those little light bulbs above their head get brighter when they finally had that eureka moment. I continued to teach the class several times when my schedule would allow, enjoying both the students and the other faculty members.

Along with teaching aspects of the regulatory system and what every manager should know, I dedicated a portion of the course to leadership and styles of management. The best aspect of leadership is to lead by example. When he taught at

West Point, President Dwight D. Eisenhower gave a demonstration to the class on real leadership. He placed a string on the table and pushed it with his finger. Nothing happened. When he pulled the string, the rest of the string followed, demonstrating that if you want people to follow you, you need to be at the head leading the charge. The students could understand this visual example.

My twin sister, Loretta, however, had a different philosophy regarding management. She believed that as a manager, there are only two things you need to know: "Whose ass to kick and whose ass to kiss." She thought most management decisions fell into those two categories. While that might be true, I also taught other methods.

I covered confidentiality when disciplining an employee. Privacy is an issue. An employee should never be corrected in front of others, an act embarrassing both to the manager and the employee. Corrections should be made in private with the emphasis on *what* was wrong rather than *who* was wrong. This eliminates a lot of potential issues with discrimination.

As a manager, when you delegate, you must supervise. Competency will always be an issue in any situation. Guaranteeing that employees understand the expectations eliminates guesswork and errors. If you lead by example, in a non-threatening manner, the employees are more apt to adhere to your expectations when you are not around.

CHANGING STUDENTS' LIVES

My students had a first-hand opportunity to observe these concepts. One young nursing unit manager often corrected her staff in the middle of the hallway or would have them walk with her while she berated them. There was no privacy. The employees often, when they saw her, would hide in the patient's room to avoid speaking with her because they never knew what she would say. I saw this as a bad example for my students.

I attempted to talk to her about her management style. She was greatly offended and stated she was in a master's program and knew full well how to manage. Little did she know at the time that in her next class at the university, I would be her professor. She was horrified when she walked into my classroom. I was nice; I did not use her as an example of how not to manage and continued with my usual lecture. She finally understood how her staff perceived her management style: as a bully or dictator. So many nurses left her unit because she did not treat them with the respect they much deserved. With knowledge comes an opportunity to change. She changed and finished her master's program. Hopefully, she put her education to use evaluating and improving her management style.

One Hispanic student in my class had difficulty writing papers. She was knowledgeable and frequently participated in class discussions. But English was a challenge. I mentored her through some books I've acquired for English as a second language to help her get her thoughts on paper in a concise and organized manner. She did very well with my mentoring sessions, and by the time she finished the class, she was on her way to becoming an excellent writer. When I ran into her several years later, she informed me she had completed her legal studies and was focusing her legal practice in immigration law. She was grateful for my help, and I was grateful for the opportunity to change her life.

I continued to teach at both the University, when time allowed, and at County Community College District. I enjoyed the students and their thirst for knowledge. Some challenged me, and I did not always have the answers. But I knew where to find them and encourage students to explore various avenues to acquire the knowledge they sought. I enjoyed sharing my stories, my experiences, and my familiarity with the students. I was honored to be the Grand Marshall at the graduation ceremonies at County Community College District. The administration warned me to stick to the script written by the program director, knowing my ability to occasionally ad-lib. It was an exciting event and brought closure to many years of dedicated teaching. A few years later, I retired, having many wonderful memories of my experiences in academia.

Chapter Eighteen:

Defending the Profession

"What cruel mistakes are sometimes made by benevolent men and women in matters of business about which they can know nothing and think they know a great deal."

— Florence Nightingale

Consulting Expert for Nursing

Early in my career around 1995, the staff of a Peer Review Organization asked me to look at documentation by a nurse and opine if the standard of care was met. At the time, I was not aware this organization looked at nursing licensure and had substantial ties to the Disciplinary Committee of the Board of Nursing. The standard of practice for nurses is usually guided by the Nurse Practice Act, which differs from state to state. In my state, Michigan, nurses worked under the guidelines of the Michigan Public Health Code, which in some areas was gray regarding the scope of practice.

In the early days of nursing, nurses did whatever doctors told them to do without question. Whether this was considered as part of nursing practice or not was questionable. In today's healthcare environment, there are many educational opportunities available to nurses to improve their hands-on skills in performing certain procedures. It would be impossible to list all the things that nurses did at the bedside and to patients. There were several attempts to develop a Nurse Practice Act in Michigan, but this was almost an impossible task.

The American Nurses Association sets the Scope and Standards of Practice (American Nurses Association , 2015) for all nurses regardless of the work environment. This describes a competent level of nursing care, as demonstrated by the critical thinking model known as the nursing process.

The Standards of Practice are as follows:

- **Standard 1. Assessment**

  The registered nurse collects pertinent data and information relative to the healthcare consumer's health or the situation.

- **Standard 2. Diagnosis**

  The registered nurse analyzes the assessment data to determine actual or potential diagnoses, problems, and issues.

- **Standard 3. Outcome Identification**

  The registered nurse identifies expected outcomes for a plan individualized to the healthcare consumer or the situation.

- **Standard 4. Planning**

  The registered nurse develops a plan that prescribes strategies to attain expected, measurable outcomes.

- **Standard 5. Implementation**

  The registered nurse implements the identified plan.

- **Standard 5A. Coordination of Care**

  The registered nurse coordinates care delivery.

- **Standard 5B. Health Teaching and Health Promotion**

  The registered nurse employs strategies to promote health and a safe environment.

- **Standard 6. Evaluation**

  The registered nurse evaluates progress toward attainment of goals and outcomes.

In addition, the American Nurses Association also set the Standards of Professional Performance (American Nurses Association, 2015) which are designed to describe a competent level of behavior in the professional role and are as follows:

- **Standard 7. Ethics**

  The registered nurse practices ethically.

- **Standard 8. Culturally Congruent Practice**

  The registered nurse acts in a manner that is congruent with cultural diversity and inclusion principles.

- **Standard 9. Communication**

  The registered nurse communicates effectively in all areas of practice.

- **Standard 10. Collaboration**

  The registered nurse collaborates with the healthcare consumer and other key stakeholders in the conduct of nursing practice.

- **Standard 11. Leadership**

  The registered nurse leads within the professional practice setting and the profession.

- **Standard 12. Education**

  The registered nurse seeks knowledge and confidence that reflects current nursing practice and promotes futuristic thinking.

- **Standard 13. Evidence-based Practice and Research**

  The registered nurse integrates evidence and research findings into practice.

- **Standard 14. Quality of Practice**

  The registered nurse contributes to quality nursing practice.

- **Standard 15. Professional Practice Evaluation**

  The registered nurse evaluates one's own and others' nursing practice.

- **Standard 16. Resource Utilization**

  The registered nurse utilizes appropriate resources to plan, provide, and sustain evidence-based nursing services that are safe, effective, and fiscally responsible.

- ## Standard 17. Environmental Health

  The registered nurse practices in an environmentally safe and healthy manner.

Not all nurses seem to be aware of the standards set by the American Nurses Association. When those standards are deviated from, situations occur that may impact the nurse's license to practice or may lead to litigation.

Every state has a State Nursing Board of Nursing that regulates and monitors nursing practice outcomes and functions through a disciplinary subcommittee that addresses performance issues. Once a complaint is made to the Board of Nursing, it is investigated and sent to an expert to evaluate whether there was a breach in the standard of practice or scope of practice. The results of that investigation are conveyed to the disciplinary subcommittee for action. Those investigations may be completed by nurses in some states, or by individuals who are trained in what to review and how to ask the right questions.

The nurse must respond to the allegations and has an opportunity for a hearing to express her side of the allegation. The Department of the Attorney General will cite the allegations against the nurse and will provide the nurse with an opportunity to respond in a timely manner. The nurse has a right to counsel and to a hearing before an Administrative Law Judge who offers his or her opinion whether the allegations were substantiated according to the letter of the law.

That report is sent to the Disciplinary Subcommittee of the Board of Nursing, who has the final say in the disciplinary process. The process may differ from state to state, but some form of action against an allegation must prevail for the sake of the safety of the community. That action may be in the form of a refresher course, limitations of practice, suspension, or revocation of the nursing license, or monetary fines.

I reviewed many cases and offered my opinions as to whether the allegations of a breach of standard of care were substantiated based on the results of the investigation. Often the nurse was not wrong but under certain circumstances took the only action that seemed safe and reasonable.

If the nurse requested a hearing, I would appear as an expert witness on behalf of the state of Michigan and with the Department of the Attorney General. My job was to explain to the Administrative Law Judge what happened, what should have happened, and where the breach in the standard of care occurred. An attorney represented the nurse to present his or her side of the issues. Since many attorneys and nurses are not familiar with the standard of practice as cited by the American Nurses Association, this complicated the defense. My role was to identify the facts. I based my opinions not on the nurse's personality but his or her actions or lack thereof.

I reviewed a case involving a nurse who was working in a teaching hospital caring for a patient who had kidney issues. The patient was sent to interventional radiology for a kidney biopsy. When the patient returned to the room, the nurse took the patient's vital signs and spoke with the family at the bedside. When she repeated the vital signs, she noticed the blood pressure was a little low. So, she repeated the blood pressure approximately every fifteen minutes, noting a downward trend. She called the radiologist to advise him of her observations, but since he was in a procedure, she was unable to speak with him. She remained at the bedside and continue to take the patient's blood pressure. This was a teaching hospital, and she made no efforts to contact the attending physician or a resident on the service. The patient went into cardiac arrest and died.

The autopsy revealed nearly three litters of blood in the abdomen due to a lacerated major vein near the kidney during the biopsy. Had this nurse contacted the resident or attending physician, the patient might have been taken immediately to surgery, and the laceration repaired. Instead, the nurse monitored the patient to death. The family however, felt the nurse was attentive and praised her efforts despite the outcome. The nurse offered no excuse for not contacting the attending or resident but claimed she thought she needed to continue monitoring the patient. The charge nurse on the unit was never involved in the care nor notified of the downward trend in the patient's blood pressure.

Another incident involved a nurse who had worked 3 to 11 shift and due to a lack of staff, was asked to work a double shift on the same unit. This happens occasionally, and if the nurses feel capable of fulfilling that assignment, they will often agree. The nurse was already familiar with the patients. A critical patient was in a room directly across the nurses' station and required multiple nursing interventions, including monitoring IV and tube feedings. The patient was in the end stage of life and not expected to survive more than the next day or so.

The wife filed the allegation against the nurse for not notifying her when her husband expired at approximately 5 AM. It was the nurse's role to contact the physician and the family when the death occurred, in addition to documenting the scenario. This nurse had extensive documentation identifying her presence at the patient's bedside, checking the IV, checking the tube feeding, and turning the patient at least every two hours. She made her last entry at 6 AM, documenting the patient as asleep and comfortable. However, that was not the case.

What the nurse didn't know was that the hallway was equipped with an ongoing video camera. I saw the video, the medical records, and interviews. The video showed the nurse taking report at the nurses' station at approximately 11:30 PM, and at about midnight, the video identified the same nurse with a pillow and a blanket walking down a dark hallway where there were multiple empty rooms. It also showed the patient's room being entered several times, almost on an hourly basis, by the patient care associate/nurse's aide. The aide, not the nurse, observed the patient.

The nurse insisted on a hearing to clear her name. She was not aware of the videotape. During that process, the Administrative Law Judge viewed the tape as did everyone else. The nurse had no explanation for her walking down the hall with a blanket and pillow since there were no patient rooms occupied on that hallway, just empty rooms. The nurse was terminated by the hospital for the falsification of medical records and dereliction of duty. She was also sanctioned by the Board of Nursing, the results of which were confidential.

Another compelling case involved a nurse working the midnight shift in a private residence caring for a five-year-old severely retarded child. The nurse's role was to monitor the tube feeding and the respiratory status of the child. The nurse knew the mother; the mother felt her child was in good hands. As the night progressed, the child needed a diaper change. Being five years old and at times combative, the child kicked the nurse several times during an attempt to change the diaper. Rather than attempting to calm the child, the nurse slapped the child on the butt hard enough to leave a handprint still identifiable in the morning. The nurse showed the mother the mark and told her the child was completely out of control. The mother took a photograph of the child's buttocks and reported the incident to the Board of Nursing for investigation.

I received the file and the photograph. To strike a retarded five-year-old child who was probably terrified in the middle of the night, to me, was unconscionable. The case went for a hearing. The nurse was represented by an aggressive attorney who insisted that nurses frequently slap patients, for instance, in trying to access a vein for an IV start. Her comparisons were ridiculous. I don't know of any nurse who would slap a patient hard enough to leave a mark for over twelve hours just to access a vein for starting an IV.

During my testimony, I was asked what the nurse should have done in that situation. I simply said the family was in the house and down the hallway. I testified she could have obtained the help of either of the patients or held the child until the child relaxed. No child ever died of a wet diaper.

The Disciplinary Subcommittee of the Board of Nursing sanctioned the nurse. It restricted her license to "no nursing contact with pediatric patients or the elderly" due to the nurse's temperament issues. She was advised to take anger management classes.

I was fair in my evaluations and based my opinions on the facts as they were presented in any case I reviewed. When the nurse was wrong, I looked for extenuating circumstances that justified his or her actions and how that impacted the standard of care.

I was soon approached by a defense attorney to look at a medical malpractice case and give my opinion on whether the standard of care was upheld. I was aware of the process and accepted the challenge of assisting him in this interesting case. That led to many opportunities to review and opine.

Legal Nurse Consulting

One of the case managers I've worked with had a husband whose best friend was an attorney, Mr. Jones, who worked for a very large law firm specializing in medical malpractice cases. This was during the time I was working for the Waterford Center and traumatic brain injury patients. This case was a perfect fit for my experience and knowledge base. Mr. Jones asked if I would review the records and give him an opinion on whether the standard of care was met on behalf of the plaintiff (the one bringing forth the legal action). "Why not?" I thought, "I am certified as a legal nurse consultant and interested in the forensic aspects of case review, looking at why things happened and what could have or should have been done to prevent certain situations." I was excited to get started.

This specific case involved a sixteen-year-old girl recuperating from a traumatic brain injury. She and her father were very close, and he was at her bedside every day. She was admitted in a comatose state and was progressing to where she would respond and started to look and smile at her dad. Although recovery was slow, she was on her way. The father and staff were encouraged by her progress.

One morning during her morning bath by the nurse's aide, the aide left the room to get more towels to complete the bath. The patient was left lying on her side, and due to becoming chilled, she went into spasms and rolled her face into the pillow. By the time the aide returned, the patient did not appear to be breathing. The aide left the room and reported her findings to the patient's nurse. The nurse immediately went to the room, evaluated the patient, and called for resuscitative efforts. They were not successful, and the patient was pronounced dead. The family sued the hospital, and the case went to trial.

My involvement in this process was to evaluate what should have happened promptly and to assist with the production of trial exhibits with the aid of an artist. I read the transcripts of the nurse's aide's deposition and the nurse's deposition, along with some of the medical records. There was quite a discrepancy noted in what the nurse testified to under oath on how she found the patient and the testimony of the nurse's aide, under oath, how she left the patient. It was obvious somebody was lying.

It was challenging to create an exhibit of how the aide claimed she left the patient and how the nurse claimed she found the patient. If you believe the nurse's aides deposition, the patient would have needed to turn herself 180° to be found in the same position as described by the nurse. From the patient's diagnosis, that would be impossible. This was a typical hospital bed and there was no room to turn 180° without the assistance of someone.

The plaintiff won at trial and the jury awarded the family several million dollars. That led to several other cases I reviewed for that law firm. Occasionally after one of my depositions, the opposing counsel approached me to review a case based on my objectivity, focusing on the facts to determine whether the situation was defensible or not.

Over the years, I received cases from both plaintiff and defense attorneys. One lawyer asked me how I could work both defense and plaintiff cases. I explained to him the facts are the facts. Just because someone comes to an attorney's office and says I want to sue the hospital, the facts may not always support a breach in a standard of care. The allegation may stem from a lack of understanding of nursing care practices.

One case comes to mind where a daughter of a ninety-five-year-old patient wanted to sue the facility because she felt her mother was given an overdose of narcotics. In this case, the patient was in severe pain due to a hip injury and was ordered 1 mg of morphine. The medication was given as ordered for the patient, and the patient was monitored for any side effects. There were no immediately noted side effects. The patient fell asleep and was no longer in pain. The dose of the medication was appropriate based on the patient's size and the amount of pain she exhibited. The patient died the following day from comorbidities and the fact that she was ninety-five years old, and the body just gave out. This was difficult for the daughter to accept. Both the family physician and I talked with her until she finally agreed that more likely than not, her mom died of old age.

A defense attorney asked me to review a case from a hospital where a nurse failed to respond to a cardiac arrest. The nurse was in the room when it appeared the patient was having respiratory distress and became pulseless. Rather than calling for a Code Blue to resuscitate the patient, the nurse just stood there and did nothing. When someone was walking by asked her what was going on, they immediately called a Code Blue and attempted to resuscitate the patient, but it was too late.

The family sued, and I could not defend the nurse's lack of timely intervention. She did absolutely nothing. During the deposition, she claimed that she froze and could not move. While that may have been exactly what happened, nurses do not have that luxury and must immediately act in response to an emergency. I later found out that this nurse left nursing practice due to this incident and was pursuing a different career path. I felt sad for her, but her decision to leave was probably a good one. In this field, hindsight is usually 100%. I look at what happened and then decide what else should or could have happened. At that time, all those options may not come to mind, and the interventions often become a knee-jerk reaction based on knowledge and experience.

I always incorporated, without sharing any names, the case facts into my lecture with my students. I gave the facts of the case and asked the class, "What would you have done?" The responses were interesting—some were correct; some were very wrong. It gave me the opportunity to provide them with a glimpse of situations they may be involved in within a short period. We discussed what the nurse did and the outcome of the investigation. It was a real eye-opener for some students who were not very focused on the facts. The facts will always be the facts. It's hard to look at things objectively when you're in the situation, which may account for some of the decisions that are made.

Families often sue to get the multimillion-dollar settlements as advertised on television. Those settlements don't often happen. Jury decisions and settlements can be appealed. In several states, when a settlement is won, Medicare or Medicaid can place a lien on the settlement and is reimbursed for the care provided. This sometimes is a big surprise to families hoping to obtain a lot of money.

Cases going to trial may not result in the expected outcomes. Plaintiffs who take the case to trial may not win. Attorneys negotiate settlements with the hope of avoiding the additional expenses of trial. Juries are unpredictable. There are no guarantees of winning the case, no matter how obvious the facts may seem.

For example, I worked on a case involving an elderly resident residing in a nursing home in New Mexico. The weather was hot, and the resident opened the window because she wanted fresh air. The facility was invaded by biting red ants. When the aide went to check on the resident, she was horrified to find the patient covered with red ants. They were even crawling in and out of her nose.

The resident sustained multiple bites that required hospitalization for treatment.

The family sued the nursing facility for neglect. During the trial, evidence was presented that the nursing facility had sprayed for red ants and other insects. This was done on a regular basis and well documented. The resident was kept clean, as evidenced by good nursing documentation and the lack of problems. The facility was air-conditioned, but the resident opened the window wanting fresh air and inadvertently invited the red ants. She got a lot more than she bargained for. The jury found the resident contributed to her problems by leaving the window open, and the nursing home was not negligent.

A local case I reviewed involved an allegation against a nursing home for allowing a resident to escape. The wife placed her husband in a nursing home because she could not control his wandering and confusion due to Alzheimer's. The nursing home promised to provide a safe environment. The patient was wearing a "wander guard" bracelet that alerted the staff when he approached the door, setting off an alarm. This was during the cold weather season. The resident walked out of the facility and was found several hundred feet away in the bush, dead from exposure to the cold.

The facility argued they frequently checked the alarms, which were in working order. They also argued that the staff immediately responded to all alarms. They asserted on the day of the escape that there were no alarms.

In reviewing the records, I noted that the resident used a walker for safe ambulation and could only ambulate approximately 50 feet before needing to rest. If indeed the alarm was responded to at the time of the alert, the resident would have barely gotten past the doorway before he was seen. The jury found on behalf of the plaintiff, and the nursing home lost its case. The evidence the defense presented did not support the facts in the case.

SERVING AS AN EXPERT WITNESS

The role of an expert witness is to clarify for the trier of fact (judge or jury) the issues in the case and if the standard of care was breached or not. Whether the review is for the plaintiff or the defense, the process does not change. The facility and/or individuals receive a notice of intent, which states they are being sued and why. Either before or after the plaintiff attorney's decision to file a suit, the attorney or legal nurse consultant reviews the medical records and other pertinent information such as physician office visits, consultation notes, and sometimes billing records.

The attorney sends the medical records to an expert for review and comment as to the standard of care. The attorney hires an expert witness with the same background as the defendants. As part of information gathering during a discovery process, both the plaintiff and defense parties answer questions to clarify the events. An Affidavit of Merit or an Affidavit of Meritorious Defense is executed by the experts to support their opinions after reviewing the data. This process varies from state to state. The experts have the right to amend their opinions as the discovery process reveals other information. Depositions of the plaintiff, defendants, witnesses, and experts take place according to the state's rules.

The process of participating in the deposition or trial can be terrifying. The plaintiff attorney takes the depositions of the defendant nurses. The nurse will generally meet with the attorney representing the defendants to clarify the process of the deposition and learn what to expect. It is important for the nurse to remember to answer only the questions that are asked. If he or she does not understand the question, the nurse should ask for it to be repeated or rephrased before he or she attempts to answer. This is not the place or time to guess. Testimony is always given under oath and recorded

The defense attorney instructs nurses to tell the truth and state the facts based on memory or knowledge. It may take years after an incident for the nurse to need to appear for a deposition. The nurse may not remember all the details and depends on the documentation in the medical record.

In the trial, the questioning may be different and often references the sworn testimony given during the deposition. It looks suspicious if the nurse suddenly remembers facts at the time of trial that she did not recall during the deposition or changes her version of the facts.

If the nurse is testifying as an expert witness, the responsibility is to explain the expert's opinions to the judge and/or jury in understandable terms. The expert summarizes the facts in the case and provides opinions. The plaintiff expert witness testifies how the standard of care was breached. The defense expert witness testifies how the defendants followed the standard of care. Experts provide clear, helpful explanations so that the judge and jury can reach fair, informed decisions.

Avoiding Mistakes

It is important to remember that nurses, doctors, and other healthcare professionals are human and therefore have the potential to make a mistake.

When that occurs, the best recourse is to document what happened and obtain medical attention for the patient, if needed. If it is a potential legal issue, the nurse should refer the situation to a risk manager for root cause analysis to prevent a reoccurrence. Healthcare staff should not lie about what happened. Families understand that unexpected occurrences or mistakes can happen, but they do not know why anybody lies to cover it up.

I reviewed a case in which the cover-up was obvious. The situation involved a thirty-two-year-old young man who entered the intensive care unit after a motorcycle accident. His injuries were serious; he was unconscious, intubated, and placed on a ventilator for respiratory support. The sister came to visit every day and was concerned about her brother's condition. One day during her visit, she noticed that her brother's two front teeth were missing; his face, nose, forehead, and chin were swollen. His lip was bleeding. The sister immediately contacted the nurse and asked, "What happened?" The nurse did not reply but stated that she would get the resident to come and explain the situation.

The resident soon arrived and told the sister that this was just an extension of his injuries and was expected. The sister was very distressed and started to cry. The roommate gestured the sister to come over to the bedside, which she did. The roommate told the sister that her brother had rolled off the bed during his morning care, hit the nightstand, and pulled out his endotracheal tube, thereby losing his teeth. The sister was horrified. She decided to return with a tape recorder and hear the explanation from the resident again.

She went home, retrieved her tape recorder, and returned. With the tape recorder in her purse, she asked the resident to explain again why her brother looked different than he had yesterday. The resident gave the same explanation that this is just the aftermath of his injuries, and it was expected. She did not mention the fall. The brother expired two days later; the sister sued.

When I reviewed the case and looked at the entries documented after the fall, there was no mention other than the swelling in the missing teeth. When I looked at the x-ray, it showed a cracked sternum, which was not evident in previous x-rays taken to evaluate endotracheal tube and central line placement.

The case went to court. During the trial, the jury had an opportunity to listen to the recording and the evidence of injury caused by the fall. The resident claimed she did not want to upset the sister since her brother would die anyway. Had the staff told the sister the truth, that during care, the patient just rolled off the bed, she may have accepted the explanations since the injuries were nonintentional. But no one will ever accept a lie to cover up a mistake. When an error occurs, own it, learn from it, do not repeat it.

Documentation becomes one of the most essential tools for defense. The purpose of documentation is to communicate the patient's progress. The patient is monitored for the effects of medication and therapies. A plan of care is important based on an assessment, interventions, and anticipated results. The plan of care must be accurate, current, periodically evaluated, and adjusted. In today's electronic medical records, plans of care and documentation are often repeated and not appropriately updated.

In one interesting case I reviewed, the patient was a brittle diabetic with heel ulcers. The plan of care addressed his diabetes and the importance of preventing pressure injury since he was immobile, on bed rest, and had a high probability of incurring a pressure injury. There was documentation to support the patient was turned every two hours. There was no notation regarding elevating the heels to prevent further breakdown. It was identified in a plan of care, but not in the nurses' notes.

The patient developed severe pressure injury and gangrene of the heels. He needed bilateral below the knee amputations. At trial, the defense counsel argued the plan of care was current. I stated it was not. He insisted I point out where it was not correct. That was not difficult. The patient now was a double amputee, and the plan of care indicated that both feet should be elevated on pills to prevent the breakdown of the heels. As I pointed out, the plan was definitely not current, as the patient had no heels to elevate.

Being the Patient's Advocate - How to Keep the Doctor from Killing Your Patient

The most important role of a nurse is to be the patient's advocate. A nurse becomes the eyes and ears of the patient. Nurses have a knowledge base and need to be assertive in speaking on the patient's behalf. Nurses should not be intimidated by physicians or mid-level providers such as physician assistants (PAs) or advanced practice nurses (NP). These providers put their pants on one leg unit time, just like the nurses. If something doesn't look right or doesn't make sense, nurses must clarify it immediately. Nurses no longer blindly follow the doctor's orders. Doctors do make mistakes. Remember, the one who graduates last in medical school is still called a doctor.

For anyone in health care, it often helps to think of their relationship to the patient like the spokes of a wagon wheel. The patient is the center or hub of the wheel, and the spokes represent those who have contact with the patient. The spokes can be physicians, nurses, physical therapy, respiratory therapy, dietary department, laboratory, radiology, and all services contributing to the well-being of that patient. Like a real wagon wheel, if any of the spokes are weak, inadequate, broken, or nonfunctioning, the wheel will not turn or support the weight of the wagon. Everyone caring for the patient has the same responsibility to put forth the best efforts for the benefit of the patient. When that does not occur, the chance of the patient progressing to a state of wellness is compromised.

It can be easy to make a mistake, even though electronic medical records reduce some kinds of errors (such as misreading handwriting). In one incident, a pharmacist was completing an entry into the database from orders received on a new admission. He walked away from the computer for a minute, and another pharmacist logged in to another medical record to make a few notes and left but did not log off. When the first pharmacist returned to the computer, he thought he was on the same patient's medical record he had been working on and continued with order entry. As he read the medical orders, he inadvertently entered orders for several doses of insulin. The insulin was transcribed to the medication administration record and noted on the wrong patient's chart. There was no sliding scale to determine the dosage of insulin required based on the patient's blood sugar. Unfortunately, the patient received two doses of insulin before the error was caught. The patient developed a hypoglycemic reaction that caused permanent brain injury. There was no order for glucose monitoring on the unit, which alerted one of the nurses to question the need for insulin.

When the pharmacist realized his mistake, he was devastated. He failed to verify the patient's name on the medical record on the computer. Mistakes do happen and can happen to anyone. Everyone responsible for providing care for the patient needs to be aware of that potential and use care. The pharmacist was disciplined by the facility and continued his work with far greater attention. Sometimes painful lessons are learned the hard way.

Chapter Nineteen

Once a Nurse Always a Nurse

"Once a nurse, always a nurse. No matter where you go what you do, you can never truly get out of nursing. It's like the Mafia. You know too much."

— Deb Gaudlin, RN

Nurses Don't Retire; They Just Lose Their Patients

THE DAY CAME when I realized it was time for me to hang up my stethoscope and nursing shoes. Tragically, my husband passed away, and I lost my twin sister in the same year. I gained an appreciation for how precious life was. My husband and I were married for forty-seven years. He was my strength, and I was his rock. He was a brittle diabetic and had chronic obstructive pulmonary disease (COPD), which impacted his ability to do anything physical. The challenges of life took their toll, and he passed away. He enjoyed my stories of molding mushy student minds into nurses. It was a great ego trip. I miss him but have many memories to keep me company.

My sister was ill for many years with congestive heart failure and became my number one patient. She had multiple cardiac procedures and numerous trips to the emergency room. She was such a frequent flyer that she was on first-name basis with the local EMS squad. We both had a sense of humor inherited from my mom, who was always the life of the party. Laughter helped her cope with her multiple health problems.

When I had some health concerns, my doctor kept reminding me that my brain might be forty-six, but my anatomy was seventy-two, and it may be time to retire and enjoy my grandchildren. They will not be small forever. It was time to revisit the bucket list and do something fun. I had to agree, although reluctantly.

 I love teaching; I love my patients, and I love sharing my knowledge and experiences with future nurses. I accomplished a lot in fifty years and have plans to achieve more. For me, life isn't over. I have a new chapter beginning. My daughter defined retirement for me as a hyphenated word, re-and tired! I can't deny that it has been my life since retirement.

I continue to work as a legal nurse consultant assisting both plaintiff and defense attorneys in the litigation process. That has kept me busy with clients in thirteen states. I genuinely enjoy the forensic aspects of completing a case review and educating attorneys on the many facets of nursing practice and the nursing process. Electronic medical record reviews have become a bit demanding due to the lack of specific documentation when an incident occurs. Healthcare providers fail to recognize that there are options to the drop-down boxes available in electronic medical records. One can always comment in addition to what selections are available. Failing to do so may not provide adequate information regarding a specific situation.

LET ME FIX THAT SLING

Due to my extensive orthopedic background, I was always fascinated to observe how individuals used assistive devices for ambulation and slings. I never had a problem approaching someone in a sling and offering some assistance to adjust the sling for comfort. I showed them where that little strap on the inside of the sling was to support their thumb and keep the arm from sliding out of the sling. That used to make my family nuts, especially my husband. He asked me, "How can you go up to a stranger and fix things?" As a nurse, that's what I did for many years. I always asked first if I might fix the sling and make it more comfortable, and no one ever said, "No." They were grateful, and I was happy I could help. I did the same with canes that appeared too short or too long for the individual using it.

NEIGHBORLY CONSULTATION

From the moment my family and friends learned that I was in nursing school, they approached me to diagnose a variety of symptoms, interpret lab data, and ask for advice on what to do. Sometimes I was able to help, and sometimes I was just as clueless as the individual asking the questions. My best advice was to contact the family doctor, ask the pharmacist about medications, or if the symptoms are frustrating or worrisome, go to urgent care or the emergency room. That, however, is probably the best advice I could give someone.

Being a nurse is a special calling. I have relieved the pain and suffering of humanity and now being asked to help a friend. How can I say no? It's part of who I am. The extent to which I want to get involved in any problem is up to me. We live in a litigious society today. I am cautious because a lack of pertinent information has an impact on the advice and the results. The one asking the questions may not be divulging all the facts. I don't want to learn the lesson the hard way!

I remember when my sister and I were young, my mother would first call Elaine, who was in nursing school at the time, for advice before she called the doctor. When my children were young, mothers of their classmates often called me for advice. If I were able and appropriately assessed the situation, I would be glad to share my knowledge.

I remember one incident where my daughter's classmate showed up with a rather nasty, shallow laceration to her leg. Apparently, she stuck her foot through a glass coffee table and sustained a 2 x 4-inch gouge. It looked like someone took a potato peeler to her leg. When I removed the Band-Aid, it looked like she needed stitches. I spoke to the mother and advised her that she should take her daughter to the emergency department for stitches to repair the wound. The child's mother claimed the wound was not infected; it looked good, didn't hurt, and would heal. It did heal but left a prominent scar. Like anything else in life, you can give advice, but it doesn't have to be taken.

I was happy to help a friend of my husband's whose wife was in hospice, at home, and in the last stages of life. She was medicated for pain but had problems with pressure injury to her ears from the oxygen tubing and a large pressure ulcer on her sacral area. The pressure ulcer on her sacral area, more likely than not, was due to the body's inability to heal. At that point, her tissue was in poor condition; she was not eating, and there was nothing left to assist in the healing process.

Her husband sat at her bedside most of the day and had accepted the fact that his wife would soon die. At the time, I was working in wound care and had a surplus of donated supplies for managing a variety of skin and wound issues. I padded her ears to prevent the irritation from the tubing. I instructed her caregiver on how to reposition her, using a wedge to prevent further pressure on her lower back. Once she was positioned comfortably and the pain in her ears was relieved, she began to relax and looked more at ease. She stopped fighting the pain medication, trying to get comfortable. You could see the relief on her husband's face, which made me feel good that I was able in some small way to assist them both.

Sitting and watching someone die is never easy, but at least they are still there. Once death occurs, they are gone but not forgotten. She died a week later. I attended the funeral. It's hard to know what to say in a situation like that, but at least the husband realized that his wife's suffering was over, and she was at peace.

I plan on keeping my nursing license current. There are so many programs and conferences I plan on attending to stay up-to-date on current trends and the latest and greatest research results. I welcome the opportunity to share my experiences with anyone who will listen. The first item on my bucket list was to write the book. I did that. I hope you enjoyed joining me as I reminisce about my nursing career.

CHAPTER TWENTY

THE FUTURE OF NURSING, AS I SEE IT

"Success is no accident. It is hard work, perseverance, learning, studying, sacrifice, and most of all the love of what you are doing or learning to do."

—Pele

FOCUS ON THE BASICS, THEY DON'T CHANGE

THE ANATOMY AND physiology of the human body have not changed over the years, but it has adapted. With new surgical procedures and innovative replacements of joints and other structures, we keep our bodies in motion and increase our life expectancies. Regardless of their environment, patients need to breathe, drink, eat, and maintain circulation to vital organs. They need a safe environment in which to heal. When any of basic human needs are not met, someone needs to intervene to assist in that recovery process. That becomes the role of the healthcare team, especially the nurse who is the patient's advocate.

As a staff nurse, when I received a new admission, my first goal was to welcome the patient and introduce myself. I would then answer any immediate questions of the patient or family. Quite often in the background, I would hear a staff member comment, "Oh no, not another new patient." This does not make the patient feel wanted or comforted. Such remarks are unnecessary since, after all, the reason for the staff's presence was to take care of sick patients. I'm sure the patient would rather be somewhere else than in the hospital. The patient and family must deal with fear, anxiety, and other issues at the time of admission. The patient may be wondering, "What's wrong with me? Will I live?" Maintaining good nurse/ patient rapport assists in educating the patient and family about the disease process, answering some of those questions and allaying their fears. The patient must be aware of the plan of care and willing to participate. This is the foundation of nursing practice. Doctors diagnose and treat, and nurses educate. Patients go to the hospital for *nursing* care.

In my career, I met several doctors who were avid teachers and supported the philosophy that if the patient knows why things are important, then they will follow instructions. Unfortunately, some physicians treat the patient like a number, and not someone with feelings, psychosocial issues, and fear. Meeting the patient's basic needs means the patient can progress to the next level of acceptance. Will nurses have the time to sit at the patient's bedside and alleviate those fears and answer the questions in the future? Only time will tell.

I have been a nurse long enough to remember when only physicians inserted Foley catheters in male patients or took blood pressures. Now, there are patient care associates, who may have worked at a fast food restaurant last week, inserting Foley catheters, drawing blood for labs, starting IVs, and doing EKGs. These tasks can be taught and learned. The question becomes what can be safely delegated by a nurse to an aide and how much education the aide needs. The aide sometimes does not understand *why* to do the task, and only perceives the *how* to do the task. Not enough or too much information both have the same effect: confusion.

Roles in health care have changed and will continue to evolve into the future based on accessible and affordable health care and human need. I ponder these questions:

- Will there be a national health plan that treats the patient from the womb to the tomb at no cost?

- How would such a free healthcare system hold the patient accountable for compliance to a plan of care?

- What would be the incentive for health-care providers to improve their skills or do research if everyone is salaried at the same rate of pay with no incentives to improve for higher wages?

THE SPAN OF NURSING EDUCATION

The two major areas that will have the most impact on nursing in the future will be education and scope of practice. Early in my career, nursing education was provided through a hospital school of nursing. This was a diploma program, typically associated with a hospital. If students wanted to pursue higher education, they had to attend college courses for four years at the university level, with no credit given for prior knowledge. Or they could pursue a two-year associate degree from a community college.

In 1969, the American Nurses Association published a paper indicating the primary education required to be considered a registered nurse is that of a Bachelor of Science degree in Nursing (BSN). Fifty years later, that recommendation is still under discussion, as it discounts the value of the Associates degree programs. (Diploma programs have faded away.)

Nurses who work in Magnet Hospitals (a reward given to hospitals that meet the criteria designed to measure the strength and quality of the nursing staff) are encouraged to obtain a bachelor's degree as soon as possible once employment is secured. The rationale behind the push for a bachelors-prepared nurse is that the liberal arts segment of the education process assists the nurse in critical thinking and looking at the patient differently. The patient is not a body with a disease and a limited treatment plan. This is an individual who, being in a healthcare facility, has other psychosocial issues to deal with besides the pathophysiology of the illness.

- Who will pay the bills?

- Who will watch the children?

- How long will I need to be in this facility or required to get care?

- When can I return to work?

The nurse works with the patient, and a healthcare team, to address these questions and concerns.

Nursing is a profession. The future nurse will need to be more involved in research and see the patient as a member of a community rather than an individual in a healthcare facility. Nursing education will focus on coordinating care. Nurses will be more aware of regulatory issues, patient access to health care, and social service programs. The concepts of primary care nursing involve overseeing the patient's care in transitioning through the continuum of care.

Nursing is a profession that requires lifelong learning. Unfortunately, there is a shortage of faculty members. Universities and colleges hire nurses with master's and doctoral degrees. This demanding role requires professors to conduct research, publish, teach, and maintain clinical competence. In general, educators are poorly paid. Nurses with masters and doctoral degrees can earn far more by becoming advanced practice registered nurses (APRN).

Sadly, for some nurses, their nursing role will never be more than a job. Their limited education or commitment caps their advancement or involvement in changing the profession. There are several programs that allow the registered nurse to obtain a bachelor's degree. Online formats allow for education without disrupting a work schedule. Schools offer credit for knowledge and experience.

Nurses with master's and doctoral degrees move from the bedside to management, administration, or research. There is often not enough incentive for nurses with higher education to remain at the bedside. Nurse practitioners now specialize in many types of clinical practices, such as emergency department, pediatrics, critical care, psychiatry, trauma, neurosurgery, orthopedics, cardiology, gynecology, long term care, to name a few. I believe nurse practitioners will specialize in areas such as working with plastic surgeons, cosmetic procedures, such as laser therapy or Botox injections. We'll see more nurse practitioners entering practice because of the programs that exist, the job opportunities, the compensation, and the rewards. Patients are often more satisfied with the services of a nurse practitioner than a physician because nurses listen and educate. Nurses, by their nature, take the time to listen to the patients and educate them on how to be healthier. Nurse practitioners provide affordable care and lower the costs of health care. It is unclear if the lower costs of providing healthcare services by a nurse, rather than a physician, will be passed on to the patient.

There is an increase in men in nursing as a profession, which can lead to a variety of new nursing opportunities. I worked with many male nurses who were just as compassionate, warm, and loving as their female coworkers. It's a fact; the profession sometimes needs a little muscle in the nursing role. Many male nurses select the emergency room, psychiatry, anesthesia, orthopedics, and the OR where being able to lift patients is essential. They may develop new roles in nursing based on their abilities and interests. Nursing has moved on from being "the sisterhood." In fact, the first male nurses were recognized during the Crusades for caring for the wounded. The future for male nurses is endless.

YOUR NEW DOCTOR-THE FUTURE SCOPE OF PRACTICE

Today when you enter an emergency room or urgent care setting for care, you may be treated by a physician's assistant (PA) or an advanced practice registered nurse (APRN). The need for safe and affordable care requires rethinking the roles of many healthcare professionals. The physician's role may change to focus on more complex cases or specialization such as ophthalmology, surgery, orthopedics, and other specialties. Nurses and physician's assistants will not replace the physician. Telemedicine and virtual intensive care units successfully stretch specialty care and offer convenience to the patient. We'll see an increase in telemedicine via cell phones, tablets, and computers.

One of health care's challenges is the disparity of regulations regarding what a mid-level provider such as an APRN can do for the patient. Many states have different rules and guidelines as to the competency and credentialing of nurse practitioners. Many exceptionally well prepared and trained nurses can't apply their skills and knowledge base due to regulations that limit their ability to perform as trained. Physician associations are vocal about what they believe nurse practitioners should do in their state. This new role of advanced practice threatens some physicians who believe advanced practice nurses may affect the physicians' professional and economic position. The general population is aging. There are not enough physicians in a primary care role to meet the needs of the aging population. Patient loads will dramatically increase as more individuals gain insurance coverage and live longer.

Prescriptive authority, admitting privileges, and ordering diagnostic tests by a nurse practitioner may vary from state to state. For example, in some states, a nurse practitioner may order medications for a patient. In others, this is prohibited. Some states allow a nurse practitioner to set up a practice without any type of collaborative relationship with a physician. Others require a physician to oversee the nurse practitioner's care.

The way I see it, knowledge is knowledge! If a physician can learn about pathophysiology and how to treat a diseased body, so can a nurse.

Nurses who have doctoral degrees (in some states, it is the essential requirement for advanced practice) are not allowed to use the title Dr. even though they earned it.

There is a lot of effort in some states to remove the barriers to the scope of practice for nurse practitioners. I feel the real emphasis needs to be a national standardization of education requirements, certification, and licensure that better defines the role of an advanced practice nurse. I believe nurses in the future will have the freedom to use their skills in providing safe and effective patient care.

Entrepreneurship and Beyond

The opportunity for nurses to be entrepreneurs or politicians exists and will change the future of nursing as well. When I began my nursing career, I had three job opportunities.

- If I was a good nurse, I worked in a hospital.

- If I was not great, I could work in a nursing home.

- If I had a great personality, I could work in an office as the physician's right hand.

Those typical nursing roles changed over the years, and the opportunities for nurses today are literally endless.

A friend of mine, who is a master's prepared nurse, had a desire to relieve patient's pain. There was no such position available in the hospital; the anesthesia department managed pain. Jessica approached senior management with the idea of having a nurse specializing in pain management working under the direction of the anesthesia department. She would take some of the workload off the anesthesia department and would have the time to monitor her patients more closely. A pain management nursing specialist would take the time to educate patients about non-medication means of pain management. Jessica successfully created her position and had time to round on patients and manage pain medication. The patients and the anesthesia department appreciated her services. Not only did she work with hospice patients, she also worked with all postoperative patients and patients who were unsuccessful in managing their chronic pain. Jessica was able to take the time to determine where the issues were and help to resolve them.

Another one of my nursing colleagues, Elizabeth, practiced Thanatology. Thanatology is the practice of studying death and the dying process. (This interest is also referred to as an end of life doula, a role assumed by some people without medical training.) She was not a morbid person, but felt patients need to be assisted through the dying process and accepting death. She visited patients who had a terminal diagnosis and helped them accept that diagnosis. She offered support so they could speak about a terminal disease to their families and proceed to a peaceful death. Over the years, some of the patients I cared for looked forward to dying and thereby ending their pain and suffering; others were terrified of the unknown.

Elizabeth was the bridge between the dead and the living. She created her position working with the chaplaincy at the hospital and the medical staff. Patients, families, and staff appreciated, accepted, and valued her services.

A motivated, persistent, and skilled nurse can create a position in a receptive environment. There will always be sick people and a need for somebody to take care of them. Jessica's and Elizabeth's jobs did not exist until they created them.

We cannot accurately foresee how nursing will evolve in the future. Patients will always need someone to care for them, someone who is warm and educated. I believe resources will be readily available at the fingertips of the nurse through electronic media devices. Robots will not replace nurses. Manufacturing companies couldn't make a robot to fulfill all the expectations placed on any nurse in any environment. Nurses today have the reputation of being able to do so much with so little that they can do just about anything with nothing.

As I write this book, there are already many designated levels of nursing practice and opportunities. The future will hold many more developed *by* nurses *for* nurses with a focus on the patient's journey from illness to health. I saw those new paths grow and participated in some of that development. I am proud of my accomplishments.

Nursing is a calling. It is not for everyone. If you are interested in nursing or other healthcare-related opportunities, volunteer in a hospital and observe those roles. Talk to healthcare providers. How do they see their role in the future? Are they satisfied with their career choice? Ask if they could change one thing in their professional role, what would it be? The answer to those questions will assist you in deciding your future.

Nursing has been kind to me over the years. I often learned as much from my patients and students as I taught them. I loved every aspect of my many nursing adventures. There is no greater feeling than helping those in need. Nursing is my passion! I hoped by sharing my stories, I have encouraged someone to explore the field of nursing. Future opportunities for nurses are endless. Welcome to my world!

Reference

American Nurses Association. (2015). *Nursing scope and standards of practice* (3rd ed.). American Nurses Association. http://www.Nursesbooks.org.

Shocking Stories of Nursing: Memoirs of a 50-year Nursing Career

Laura A. Conklin, MSN, MSA, RN, President

Conklin and Associates, LLC

Nurlewood Publishing, LLC

21718 Edgewood St.

St. Clair Shores, MI 48080

laconklin2000@yahoo.com

Cell Phone: (586) 596-5239

Home Phone: (586)776-0117

Fax: (586) 776-0118

PLEASE WRITE A REVIEW

When you enjoy a book, it is a natural desire to tell others about it. Amazon.com provides a way to share your thoughts and I invite you to write a book review. It is easy. Here are tips:

1. Do a search in Amazon.com by going to books, using Laura A. Conklin. The first thing you are asked to do is to **assign several stars** to the book you think matches your opinion of the book.

2. Create a **title** for the review. This can be a simple phrase, like "Awesome Tip Book." If you are not sure what to say, look at the titles of other book reviews.

3. It is easiest to write the book in a **word processor** and then paste it into Amazon.com. Your word processor will pick up typos before your review goes public.

4. Write the review as if you were **talking to another person** – you are – a person who comes to Amazon.com and is considering buying this book.

5. Include a description of what you found **most helpful**. Was it an idea, chapter, tip? Share that with the readers.

6. Next you may want to write **who you think would most benefit** from this book. Is it for beginners? Or is it more appropriate for some- one with experience with this topic?

7. What if you have something **negative** to say about the book? You may always reach me at laconklin2000@yahoo.com to suggest changes in the book.

8. If you include negative feedback in the review, keep a positive perspective rather than attack me.

Here are some sample phrases:
- While overall the book was good, I would change it by…

- I don't think this book is right for. . .

- I would improve this book by. . .

Before you hit save, **read everything over one more time**. Authors and readers appreciate book reviews and they get easier to write with time.

Also please email me at laconklin2000@yahoo. com when you have posted your review.

Thank you,

Laura A. Conklin